Nail Technician and Nail Reconstruction

A Practical Guide to Mastering All Techniques and Becoming a Professional!

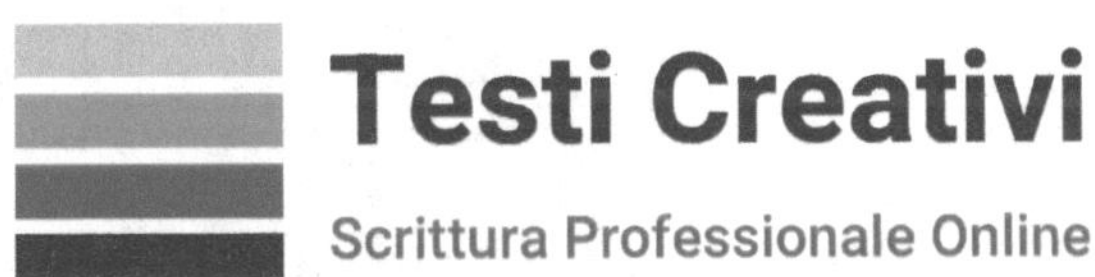

Indice

🎁 **At the end of this book you'll find an exclusive gift!**

13

Nail Technician and Nail Reconstruction

A Practical Guide to Mastering All Techniques and Becoming a Professional!

I. Introduction to Nail Technology

1. Origins and Evolution of Nail Technology

The craft of nail care, also known as nail technology, has deep roots in ancient civilizations. From the earliest times, people have placed importance on the care and aesthetics of nails, not only as a sign of beauty but also as an indicator of social status and personal well-being. In ancient Egypt, aristocratic women painted their nails with natural pigments, while in China, long, well-maintained nails were a symbol of wealth and nobility. Over the centuries, nail care and decoration techniques have evolved, reflecting the trends and traditions of various cultures.

However, it was in the 20th century that nail technology underwent a true revolution. With the advent of mass production and the proliferation of cosmetic products, people began exploring new possibilities for nail care and embellishment. In the 1950s, the popularity of artificial nails and colored nail polishes ushered in a new era in the nail industry.

In the following years, with technological advancements and the growing demand for more durable and natural treatments, techniques for nail reconstruction using gel, acrylic, and acrigel emerged. These materials, initially developed for medical purposes, quickly found applications in nail aesthetics, offering a long-lasting solution for strengthening and decorating natural nails.

Today, nail technology has become a profession in its own right, with specialized technicians offering a wide range of services, from simple manicures to advanced nail reconstruction. With access to professional training and high-quality materials, anyone can learn nail reconstruction techniques and embark on a rewarding career in the nail aesthetics industry.

2. The Role of Nail Reconstruction Techniques

Nail reconstruction techniques using gel, acrylic, and acrigel play a fundamental role in the nail aesthetics industry, offering innovative solutions to address a range of aesthetic and functional issues. These techniques not only enhance the appearance of nails but also aim to improve their health and strength.

One of the primary functions of reconstruction techniques is to strengthen natural nails, especially for individuals with brittle nails that tend to break easily. Due to the resilience and durability of gel, acrylic, and acrigel, it is possible to protect natural nails from harmful external factors such as moisture and impacts, thus preventing breakage and damage.

Additionally, these techniques allow for the correction of structural nail defects, such as onycholysis (the separation of the nail from the nail bed), damaged, or deformed nails. By using gel, acrylic, or acrigel, nails can be uniformly shaped, creating a smooth and even surface that enhances the overall appearance of the hands.

However, reconstruction techniques are not limited to reinforcement and correction functions. They also offer endless creative possibilities for nail art. With the use of colored gels, glitter, gems, and other decorations, unique and personalized designs can be created that express each client's personality and style. From elegant French manicures to bolder and more imaginative designs, reconstruction techniques allow technicians to showcase their creativity and meet diverse aesthetic needs.

Moreover, reconstruction techniques provide solutions for specific nail issues, such as nail-biting or nails damaged by chemical treatments. By fully covering the natural nail with durable materials, it is possible to protect damaged nails during the growth process, allowing them to regenerate in a safe and protected environment.

In conclusion, nail reconstruction techniques with gel, acrylic, and acrigel are a valuable resource for anyone looking to improve the appearance and health of their nails. With proper training and practice, technicians can use these techniques to offer high-quality services and meet the needs of their most demanding clients.

3. Career Opportunities in Nail Technology

Nail technology is not just a skill to possess but also a profession that offers a wide range of career opportunities. With the growing awareness of the importance of nail care and the increasing demand for beauty and wellness services, the need for qualified technicians is continually rising. This means that anyone with expertise in nail technology has multiple pathways to professional success.

One of the most common career paths in nail technology is working as a technician in a beauty salon or a specialized nail studio. In these settings, technicians have the opportunity to serve a diverse clientele, offering a variety of treatments, from basic manicures to advanced nail reconstruction. Working in a professional environment allows technicians to gain practical experience and build a reputation in the industry.

Other technicians choose to start their own business as entrepreneurs in the nail aesthetics sector. This can mean opening their own beauty salon, offering mobile services, or even selling nail technology products and materials. With the right planning and marketing, it is possible to create a successful business and earn a loyal clientele.

But career opportunities in nail technology are not limited to traditional beauty salons. With the advent of technology and the digital world, more and more technicians are exploring new ways to offer their services online. Through social media platforms, blogs, and video tutorials, it is possible to reach a wide audience of potential clients and build a personal brand in the nail aesthetics industry.

Additionally, nail technology also offers career opportunities in the field of teaching and training. With the experience and skills acquired over time, technicians can become certified instructors and share their knowledge with other aspiring technicians. This not only contributes to the growth and development of the industry but also offers a rewarding opportunity for mentorship and leadership.

In conclusion, career opportunities in nail technology are varied and exciting. With dedication, training, and practice, anyone with a passion for nail care can find success and professional fulfillment in this rapidly growing field.

4. Purpose and Content of the Manual

This manual has been created with the aim of providing a comprehensive overview of advanced nail reconstruction techniques using gel, acrylic, and acrigel, offering both beginners and advanced users a detailed and practical guide to mastering this fascinating profession in the nail aesthetics field.

The content of the manual is structured in a logical and progressive manner, starting from the fundamental basics and moving towards more advanced techniques. Each chapter is designed to be accessible and comprehensible, with detailed instructions, explanatory images, and practical tips to ensure a complete understanding and effective application of the techniques illustrated.

We begin by exploring the basic concepts of nail technology, opening the doors to aspiring technicians and introducing them to the wonderful world of nails. Subsequently, we delve into the various reconstruction techniques using gel, acrylic, and acrigel, providing step-by-step instructions on how to prepare the natural nail, apply the materials, and finish the work to achieve professional results.

However, this manual is not limited to the practical aspects of these techniques. We will also address crucial issues such as hygiene and safety, offering practical advice on how to maintain a clean and safe workstation and protect both the technician and the client from potential risks of infection or damage.

Additionally, we will dedicate space to solving common problems that may arise during nail technology practice, offering practical solutions and tips to avoid mistakes and improve skills over time.

Finally, the manual will include useful tips for maintaining reconstructed nails, marketing and promoting nail technician services, as well as a reflection on the future prospects of this ever-evolving profession.

In summary, our goal with this manual is to provide aspiring technicians with a broad knowledge of nail reconstruction techniques using gel, acrylic, and acrigel, equipping them with the skills and knowledge necessary to excel in this exciting profession within the nail aesthetics industry.

5. Exploring the Possibilities of Nail Technology

Nail technology offers a world of creative and professional possibilities that extend far beyond simply applying nail polish and decorations. With the right training and practice, technicians can explore a wide range of services and specializations, meeting diverse needs of their clients and making a mark in the nail aesthetics industry.

One of the primary opportunities that nail technology provides is the ability to create unique and personalized designs that reflect each client's style and personality. Using colored gels, glitter, gems, stickers, and other decorations, technicians can transform nails into works of art, creating looks that range from simple elegance to bold fantasy.

However, the possibilities of nail technology are not limited to nail decoration alone. Technicians can also specialize in nail care and treatment services, offering solutions for specific issues such as weak, damaged, or fungal-infected nails. By employing reinforcement and reconstruction techniques using gel, acrylic, or acrigel, it is possible to enhance the health and resilience of natural nails, allowing them to grow healthy and strong over time.

Furthermore, nail technology offers opportunities for career expansion through training and specialization in related fields. For instance, many technicians choose to broaden their skills by learning 3D nail art techniques, nail stamping, or nail piercing. Others opt for specialization in more advanced treatments such as acrylic nails adorned with Swarovski crystal embellishments or ombre-effect nail extensions.

Moreover, nail technology can also open doors to employment opportunities in related industries such as fashion, entertainment, and marketing. With the rising popularity of nail influencers and world-renowned nail technicians, there is an increasing demand for qualified technicians who can create innovative and eye-catching looks for special events, fashion shows, film productions, and advertising campaigns.

In conclusion, exploring the possibilities of nail technology means delving into a world of creativity, innovation, and professional opportunities. With passion, dedication, and proper training, anyone with a love for nail care can find success and fulfillment in this ever-evolving field.

II. Necessary Tools and Materials

1. Files: Essential Tools for Nail Shaping

Files are among the most fundamental tools in a nail technician's arsenal, playing a crucial role in shaping, refining, and defining the nail's form. Choosing the right file can make the difference between a well-executed job and a disappointing result, so it's important to understand the various types available and learn how to use them correctly.

There are various types of files, each with specific characteristics suited to different shaping needs. Fine-grit files are ideal for refining and smoothing nails, ensuring a smooth and even surface without damaging the nail bed. Conversely, more abrasive files are used to quickly and effectively reduce nail length and shape, but it's essential to use them carefully to avoid excessive damage.

For nail shaping, it's advisable to use rectangular or curved files, depending on personal preference and the type of work being done. Rectangular files offer greater precision and control in defining the shape, while curved files better conform to the natural curvature of the nails, making shaping and smoothing easier.

When using files, it's important to pay attention to the direction and pressure applied, avoiding abrupt movements and excessive abrasion that could damage natural nails. It's recommended to file in one direction, back and forth, maintaining even pressure to achieve a uniform and professional result.

Furthermore, keeping files clean and well-maintained is important for optimal performance and to prevent contamination or infections. After each use, it's advisable to clean files with water and mild soap or a specific disinfectant for nail tools, and store them in a clean, dry container to prevent contamination from bacteria or fungi.

In conclusion, files are essential tools for nail shaping and refining, offering precision, control, and versatility in the processing. With the correct selection and use of files, it's possible to achieve professional results and meet the diverse aesthetic needs of clients.

2. Buffers: Smoothing and Preparing Nails for Reconstruction

The buffer is an indispensable tool in every nail technician's toolkit, used to smooth and prepare the natural nail before reconstruction with gel, acrylic, or acrigel. Its abrasive action helps eliminate surface irregularities, creating a uniform and adhesive base for the application of reconstructive materials. However, using the buffer correctly requires careful attention and technique to avoid damage to the natural nails and ensure optimal results.

There are various types of buffers available on the market, each with specific features suited to different processing needs. Fine-grit buffers are ideal for gently smoothing the surface of the natural nail, preparing it for reconstruction without damaging the nail bed. Conversely, more abrasive buffers can be used to remove the superficial layer of the nail, ensuring better adhesion of reconstructive materials.

During the use of the buffer, it's important to pay attention to the applied pressure and the direction of movements, avoiding excessive force or over-filing. The correct technique involves light and fluid movements, keeping the buffer flat to avoid excessive damage to the nail surface. Additionally, it's advisable to use the buffer only on the nail plate and avoid filing near the cuticles or soft parts of the skin to prevent irritation or injury.

After buffing the nail, it's crucial to carefully remove dust residues and clean the surface with a dehydrator or primer to enhance the adhesion of reconstructive materials. This preparatory step is essential to ensure optimal and long-lasting adherence of the reconstruction, avoiding premature lifting or detachment.

In conclusion, buffers are versatile and essential tools in the practice of nail technology, offering the ability to smooth and prepare the natural nail for reconstruction with gel, acrylic, or acrigel. With proper technique and attention to detail, nail technicians can achieve professional results and effectively meet the aesthetic needs of their clients.

3. Brushes: Precision Tools for Gel, Acrylic, and Acrygel Application

Brushes are indispensable in every nail technician's toolkit, playing a crucial role in the precise and uniform application of gel, acrylic, and acrygel. The choice of the right brush can significantly influence the quality of the finished work, so it's essential to understand the various characteristics of available brushes and how to use them effectively.

There are different types of brushes, each designed to meet specific needs during the application process of reconstructive materials. Gel brushes are generally softer and more flexible, with thin and smooth bristles that allow for even distribution of gel on the natural nail. These brushes are particularly suitable for creating thin layers of gel and executing detailed nail art decorations.

On the other hand, acrylic brushes are typically firmer and more robust, with denser and compact bristles that enable greater precision and control. These brushes are ideal for acrylic application, allowing technicians to easily shape and mold acrylic on the nail surface, creating custom shapes and designs.

Acrygel brushes offer a hybrid option, designed to provide the versatility of gel with the strength of acrylic. These brushes feature softer bristles compared to acrylic brushes, but they are stiffer than gel brushes, allowing technicians to work effectively and precisely with both materials. They are particularly suitable for the acrygel technique, which combines gel and acrylic for enhanced durability and strength.

During the use of brushes, it's important to pay attention to cleaning and maintenance to ensure optimal performance and prolonged lifespan. After each use, brushes should be cleaned with a solvent specific to the type of material used and stored appropriately to prevent bristle deformation or contamination from product residues.

In conclusion, brushes are essential tools for achieving professional results in nail reconstruction with gel, acrylic, and acrygel. With proper selection and use of brushes, technicians can execute a wide range of techniques and designs with precision and creativity, satisfying the aesthetic needs of their clients.

4. UV/LED Lamps: Efficient Polymerization of Materials

UV/LED lamps are essential tools in the field of nail reconstruction with gel, acrylic, and acrygel, enabling rapid and efficient polymerization of the materials used. These lamps emit ultraviolet or LED light that activates the photoinitiators present in gels and acrygels, triggering the polymerization reaction that transforms the liquid materials into a solid hardened structure.

The choice between UV and LED lamps depends on personal preferences and specific technician needs. UV lamps have traditionally been used in the nail industry, offering effective polymerization of gels and acrygels. However, they require longer curing times and may pose a higher risk of skin damage due to exposure to ultraviolet rays.

On the other hand, LED lamps have become increasingly popular for their higher efficiency and excellent durability. LED lamps can polymerize materials in shorter times compared to UV lamps, reducing total working time and improving productivity. Moreover, they emit less heat and do not emit harmful ultraviolet rays, making them a safer choice for both the technician and the client.

Regardless of the type of lamp chosen, it is important to follow manufacturer instructions and adhere to recommended curing times to ensure optimal results. Proper positioning of the hands under the lamp during the polymerization process is also advisable to ensure even distribution of light and complete polymerization of materials on all nail surfaces.

Furthermore, it's important to consider the specific characteristics of the materials used. For example, some gels and acrygels may require longer curing times or may necessitate a higher-power UV or LED lamp for effective polymerization. Therefore, it is advisable to always check the manufacturer's recommendations and adjust lamp usage to the specific needs of the materials being used.

In conclusion, UV/LED lamps are essential tools for ensuring efficient polymerization of materials in nail reconstruction with gel, acrylic, and acrygel. With proper selection and use of the lamp, high-quality work can be achieved, ensuring the durability and strength of the reconstruction.

5. Primer and Dehydrator: Preparing the Natural Nail

Primer and dehydrator are essential products in preparing the natural nail before reconstruction with gel, acrylic, or acrygel. These products play distinct yet complementary roles in the preparation process, ensuring optimal adhesion of the reconstructive materials and long-term durability of the reconstruction.

Primer is an adhesive liquid applied to the natural nail before applying gel, acrylic, or acrygel. Its primary task is to enhance material adhesion by creating a stronger and more durable bond between the natural nail and the reconstructive material. Primer works by penetrating the nail's surface layers, creating a slightly rough surface that facilitates the bonding of gel or acrylic.

On the other hand, dehydrator is a product used to remove moisture and natural oils from the nail's surface, preparing it for the application of primer and reconstructive materials. Its dehydrating action helps eliminate any oil residue, dirt, or remnants of nail polish from the nail, ensuring better adhesion and longer-lasting reconstruction.

Correct application of primer and dehydrator is crucial for achieving optimal results and preventing premature lifting or detachment of the reconstruction. Before application, it's important to thoroughly prepare the natural nail by cleaning the surface with a specific cleanser or nail polish remover to remove any dirt or oil residue.

Once clean and dry, the nail can be treated with dehydrator to remove moisture and prepare the surface for primer application. After the dehydrator has dried, proceed with applying primer, ensuring it is evenly distributed over the entire nail surface and avoiding contact with the surrounding skin.

After applying the primer, it's important to allow it to dry completely before proceeding with the application of reconstructive materials. This allows the primer to create a solid and durable bond with the natural nail, ensuring better adhesion and longer durability of the reconstruction over time.

In conclusion, primer and dehydrator are essential in preparing the natural nail for reconstruction with gel, acrylic, or acrygel. With correct application and preparation, optimal results and long-term durability of the reconstruction can be achieved.

6. Gel, Acrylic, and Acrygel: Fundamental Materials for Reconstruction

Gel, acrylic, and acrygel are the three main materials used in nail reconstruction, each with unique characteristics and specific advantages. With a proper understanding and mastery of these materials, a wide range of techniques can be executed, creating customized designs to meet clients' aesthetic needs.

Gel is a versatile and flexible material, available in various consistencies and viscosities to suit technician preferences and client requirements. Gel can be used for nail extensions, reinforcement, or repairs of natural nails, allowing for greater customization and creativity in designs. One of the advantages of gel is its ability to self-level during polymerization, creating a smooth and even surface without the need for excessive filing. Gel can be polymerized with UV or LED lamps, ensuring quick and complete curing of the material.

Acrylic is a durable and resilient material widely used in nail reconstruction for its strength and resistance to breakage. Composed of a mixture of liquid polymers and monomers that quickly harden when exposed to air, acrylic allows for precise handling and detailed shaping of nails. Acrylic can be used to create nail extensions, add reinforcements, or sculpt custom shapes, offering greater strength and durability compared to gel. However, it requires careful attention during application and shaping, as it solidifies quickly and can be challenging to correct once hardened.

Acrygel represents an innovative combination of gel and acrylic, offering the best of both worlds in terms of flexibility, strength, and durability. This hybrid material allows for superior adhesion and enhanced flexibility compared to traditional gel, ensuring greater durability and resistance to nail breakage. Acrygel can be applied and sculpted using the same techniques as acrylic, providing the opportunity to create detailed and customized designs without compromising the material's durability and strength. It is cured with UV or LED lamps, ensuring complete and rapid hardening of the material for a professional and long-lasting result.

In conclusion, gel, acrylic, and acrygel are fundamental materials in the practice of nail technology, offering the opportunity to execute a wide range of techniques and create customized designs to meet clients' aesthetic needs. With a proper understanding and mastery of these materials, professional and durable results can be achieved in nail reconstruction.

7. Trays and Containers: Organization and Storage of Tools

Trays and containers are crucial elements for maintaining order and cleanliness in a nail technician's workspace. Proper organization of tools not only facilitates work during nail reconstruction but also ensures a safe and hygienic environment for both the technician and the client.

Various types of trays and containers are available on the market, each designed to meet specific needs for organizing and storing tools. Trays can be used for soaking clients' hands during manicures or gel removal, providing a comfortable and relaxing environment. Transparent containers are ideal for storing files, buffers, brushes, and other tools, allowing the technician to easily see the contents and quickly access necessary tools during work.

It's important to regularly clean and disinfect trays and containers to prevent cross-contamination and protect the health of both the client and the technician. After each use, it's advisable to clean trays and containers with water and neutral soap or with a specific disinfectant for tools to ensure effective removal of any product residue or bacteria.

Furthermore, attention should be paid to the arrangement of tools inside trays and containers to maximize efficiency and reduce the risk of contamination. For example, it's recommended to separate tools used for preparing the natural nail from those used for applying reconstructive materials, avoiding direct contact between the two phases of the process.

Proper organization of tools also contributes to creating a professional and welcoming environment for the client, demonstrating attention to detail and dedication to the work. Clients will feel more secure and confident in receiving high-quality treatments in a well-organized and clean environment.

In conclusion, trays and containers are essential tools for maintaining order, cleanliness, and safety in a nail technician's workspace. With proper organization and maintenance of tools, it's possible to ensure a professional and hygienic environment for performing high-quality treatments and meeting clients' aesthetic needs.

8. Disinfectants and Hygiene Products: Workplace Safety and Hygiene

Workplace safety and hygiene are paramount for every nail technician, as they contribute to protecting both the client's and the professional's health and preventing the spread of infections or contaminations. Disinfectants and hygiene products play an essential role in maintaining a safe and hygienic work environment, ensuring compliance with health regulations and customer satisfaction.

Disinfectants are used to eliminate germs, bacteria, and viruses from work surfaces, tools, and equipment, reducing the risk of contamination and infection. There are various types of disinfectants available, including alcohol-based disinfectants, chlorine-based, quaternary ammonium, and other antimicrobial agents. It is important to select an effective disinfectant suitable for the specific needs of the workstation, ensuring it can eliminate a wide range of pathogens without damaging treated tools or surfaces.

In addition to disinfectants, it is crucial to use personal hygiene products such as disposable gloves, face masks, and protective gowns to reduce the risk of cross-contamination between the technician and the client. These products protect the client from potential contamination by the technician and shield the technician from exposure to harmful chemicals present in products used during nail treatments.

Strict hygiene practices must be followed during all stages of nail treatment, including cleaning and disinfecting the technician's and client's hands before starting the treatment. Furthermore, it is important to regularly clean and disinfect all work surfaces, including tables, UV/LED lamps, trays, and tool containers, to prevent contamination by bacteria or other pathogens.

Finally, educating the client about the importance of hygiene and safety during nail treatment is essential, encouraging them to follow the technician's recommendations and adopt personal hygiene practices at home. This helps maintain nail health and prevents potential complications or infections after treatment.

In conclusion, the use of disinfectants and hygiene products is essential to ensure workplace safety and hygiene for a nail technician. With proper selection and use of these products, it is possible to create a safe and hygienic work environment, protecting the health of both the client and the technician and ensuring high-quality results in nail treatment.

9. Decorative Accessories: Personalizing Reconstructed Nails

Decorative accessories are a fundamental element in personalizing reconstructed nails, allowing clients to express their individuality and style through unique and creative designs. With a wide range of accessories available, including gems, rhinestones, stickers, glitter, and metal decorations, nail technicians have the opportunity to create customized and fashionable designs that meet the aesthetic needs of the client.

Gems and rhinestones are among the most popular accessories used to add a touch of brilliance and glamour to reconstructed nails. They can be applied on gel or acrylic during the modeling phase or on the nail surface after the reconstruction process, creating luminous and three-dimensional effects that capture attention. Gems come in various shapes, sizes, and colors, allowing for a wide range of creative possibilities and personalized designs.

Stickers are a quick and easy option to add designs and patterns to nails without requiring specific artistic skills. They are available in a variety of motifs, including flowers, animals, geometrics, and more, and can be applied to the nail surface after the reconstruction process. Stickers allow clients to easily change their style and look, experimenting with different designs without long-term commitment.

Glitters are perfect for adding a touch of sparkle and glamour to nails, creating bright and shiny effects that stand out. They can be incorporated into gel or acrylic during the modeling phase or applied to the nail surface after the reconstruction process, allowing clients to customize their look with luminous and brilliant reflections.

Metal decorations, such as beads, chains, and charms, add an element of elegance and sophistication to nails, creating sophisticated and fashionable designs. They can be applied to the nail surface or incorporated into gel or acrylic during the modeling phase, allowing clients to personalize their look with intricate and chic details.

In conclusion, decorative accessories offer endless possibilities for personalizing reconstructed nails, allowing clients to express their creativity and style through unique and fashionable designs. With a wide range of options available, nail technicians have the opportunity to create customized looks that meet the aesthetic needs of the client and ensure high-quality results.

10. Solvents and Gel Removers: Corrections and Cleaning During the Work Process

Solvents and gel removers are essential tools in the nail technician's work process, providing effective solutions for correcting errors, cleaning, and preparing nails during reconstruction. With a proper understanding and use of these products, it is possible to optimize efficiency and precision in work, ensuring professional and satisfying results for the client.

Solvents are used to remove residue from gel, acrylic, or acrylic-gel from the nail surface during the modeling process. They can correct application errors, clean, and prepare nails before applying new layers of reconstructive material. Solvents can be acetone-based or specific solvents tailored to the type of material used, ensuring effective removal without damaging the natural nail.

Gel removers are specially formulated to remove cured gel or gel polish from nails without damaging the nail surface. They come in various forms such as liquids, gels, or wraps, and can be applied to the nail surface to soften and dissolve excess gel. These products are particularly useful during the gel removal phase before applying a new gel layer or performing a complete nail reconstruction.

During the work process, it is important to use solvents and gel removers carefully and follow manufacturer instructions to ensure safe and effective removal of materials. It is advisable to always test the product on a small area of skin to check for any allergic reactions or irritations before full use.

Furthermore, maintaining a clean and organized workstation during the use of solvents and gel removers is crucial to avoid cross-contamination and protect the health of both the client and technician. Disposable or sterilized tools should be used to apply the products, and any excess residue should be removed with a clean cloth or cotton pad.

In conclusion, solvents and gel removers are essential tools in the nail technician's work process, enabling precise corrections and effective cleaning during reconstruction. With a proper understanding and use of these products, it is possible to ensure professional and satisfying results for the client while maintaining a safe and hygienic work environment.

III. Preparing the Workstation

1. Organization of Tools and Materials

Proper organization of tools and materials is crucial for creating an efficient and tidy workspace during the nail reconstruction process. A well-prepared nail technician can optimize their workflow and ensure greater precision and quality in the final results.

First and foremost, having a clear overview of all the necessary tools for nail reconstruction is important. These may include files, buffers, brushes for gel, acrylic, and acrylgel, spatulas, tweezers, and other specialized utensils. Ensuring all tools are readily accessible reduces time spent searching and increases process efficiency.

Once the tools are identified, it's essential to organize them systematically and accessibly. Using containers or organizers with separate compartments keeps tools separated and orderly. For instance, assigning one container for files and buffers, another for brushes and spatulas, and so on. This facilitates easy retrieval of necessary tools during treatments and reduces the risk of confusion or disorder.

Regarding materials, strategically placing them on the workstation is important. Gel, acrylic, and acrylgel should be positioned in containers or dispensers that allow easy access and precise dispensing. Additionally, storing materials in closed containers protects them from external contamination and extends their shelf life.

Lastly, maintaining a clean and tidy workstation throughout the process is crucial. Regularly removing residues of gel, acrylic, or acrylgel from work surfaces and disinfecting tools after each use is recommended. Keeping a hygienic workspace is essential for both the client's and technician's health and ensures high-quality results.

2. Sterilization of Instruments

Sterilization of instruments is a crucial aspect in the field of nail technology, ensuring an optimal level of hygiene and safety for the client. Proper sterilization of instruments is essential to prevent the transmission of infections and ensure safe and ethical working practices.

There are several methods of sterilizing instruments, each with its own advantages and limitations. One of the most effective methods is the use of an autoclave, a device that uses high-pressure steam and temperature to eliminate bacteria, viruses, fungi, and other pathogenic microorganisms. The autoclave sets the benchmark for instrument sterilization in the healthcare sector, as it can guarantee a level of sterilization certified and compliant with international standards.

In addition to autoclaving, other methods of instrument sterilization include using chemical disinfectant solutions, UV radiation, or dry heat. However, it's important to note that some of these methods may not be as effective in eliminating all pathogenic microorganisms and could pose a risk to client safety if not performed correctly.

Regardless of the method used, it is crucial to strictly follow guidelines and recommendations provided by the instrument and sterilizing material manufacturers. This includes adhering to sterilization times and temperatures, as well as using disinfectant solutions with proven efficacy against a wide range of pathogens.

Furthermore, maintaining accurate documentation of instrument sterilization activities, including detailed records of sterilization cycles and periodic inspections of instruments, is important. This not only demonstrates a commitment to safety and hygiene but may also be required by local regulations or regulatory authorities.

In conclusion, instrument sterilization is a critical process in nail technology that requires attention to detail, precision, and adherence to safety standards. Investing in best sterilization practices ensures client safety and enhances the professional reputation of the nail technician.

3. Arrangement of Reconstructive Materials

The arrangement of reconstructive materials on the workstation is a crucial element in ensuring an efficient and organized workflow during the nail reconstruction process. Each type of material, whether gel, acrylic, or polygel, requires specific attention to arrangement and accessibility to ensure proper application and optimal final results.

Regarding gel, it is advisable to have various types such as builder gel for apex construction and nail structure modeling, base gel for application on natural nails, and top coat gel for a glossy and durable finish. These gels should be stored in transparent containers or dispensers that are well-labeled for easy identification during work.

For acrylic, it's important to have different monomers and polymers available to create optimal and controlled consistency during application. Acrylics may come in various colors, viscosities, and drying times, so having a variety of options on hand is crucial to meet specific client needs and project requirements.

As for polygel, which combines aspects of both gel and acrylic, having base materials for both components and specialized polygel products like gel activator and gel cleanser is important. These materials should be arranged to allow quick and precise mixing during application to ensure a uniform and long-lasting finish.

In addition to organizing the materials themselves, it's important to consider the cleaning and maintenance of tools and containers used for reconstructive materials. Containers should be regularly cleaned and disinfected to prevent cross-contamination and protect client health. Tools such as spatulas and brushes should be cleaned after each use and stored safely to avoid damage or contamination.

In conclusion, proper arrangement of reconstructive materials is essential to ensure an efficient workflow and high-quality nail reconstruction. Investing time and effort into organizing and maintaining the workstation leads to better and more satisfying results for the client.

4. Cleaning and Sanitization of the Workstation

Cleaning and sanitization of the workstation are fundamental aspects in the practice of nail technology, as they contribute to ensuring a safe and hygienic environment for both the client and the technician. A clean and well-maintained workstation not only reduces the risk of infections transmitted by bacteria and other pathogens but also enhances the professional image and client confidence in the service provided.

Before commencing any treatment, it is important to dedicate time to cleaning and sanitizing the workstation. This includes cleaning work surfaces, material containers, tools, and any other areas or objects that may come into contact with the client or materials used during treatment.

For cleaning work surfaces, it is advisable to use mild detergents and approved disinfectants that are effective against a wide range of pathogenic microorganisms, including bacteria, viruses, and fungi. It is important to carefully follow the manufacturer's instructions to ensure safe and effective use of the products.

Regarding material containers, regular cleaning and disinfection are recommended to prevent cross-contamination between different products used during treatment. Diluted disinfectant solutions or specific cleaners suitable for plastic or glass containers can be used for this purpose.

Tools used during treatment should be cleaned and disinfected after each use to prevent transmission of infections between clients. Using an approved disinfectant solution and leaving the tools immersed for the manufacturer-recommended time ensures effective elimination of pathogenic microorganisms.

Finally, adopting rigorous personal hygiene practices such as frequent hand washing and the use of disposable gloves during treatment further reduces the risk of contamination.

In conclusion, cleaning and sanitization of the workstation are essential practices to ensure a safe, hygienic, and professional environment in the field of nail technology. Investing time and effort into these practices helps protect the health of both the client and the technician and ensures high-quality results.

5. Safety Conditions Check

Checking the safety conditions of the workstation is a crucial step to ensure a safe working environment and avoid potential risks or incidents during nail reconstruction treatments. Workplace safety is a top priority for every nail technician, and regular checks of safety conditions are essential to identify and mitigate any hazards or risky situations.

Before starting any treatment, it is important to ensure that the workstation is free of obstacles and well-lit to ensure optimal visibility during work. Additionally, it is essential to verify that all tools and materials are securely positioned and accessible, thereby reducing the risk of accidents or falls.

In addition to arranging tools and materials, it is also important to examine the maintenance and operation status of the tools and equipment used during treatment. For instance, it is critical to verify that UV/LED lamps used for curing materials are in good working condition and do not show any signs of damage or malfunction that could compromise the safety of the client and technician.

Another crucial aspect is checking the cleanliness and hygiene conditions of the workstation. Ensuring that all surfaces are clean and disinfected reduces the risk of bacterial contamination and helps maintain a safe and hygienic work environment. Furthermore, it is important to check that material containers are properly sealed and free from leaks or spills that could pose a safety hazard.

Finally, it is important to be aware of workplace safety regulations and guidelines and ensure compliance with them at every stage of the treatment. This includes the correct use of personal protective equipment such as disposable gloves and masks, and adopting safe and ethical work practices.

In conclusion, checking the safety conditions of the workstation is an essential step to ensure a safe, hygienic, and professional work environment in the field of nail technology. Investing time and effort in safety checks helps protect the health of both the client and the technician and ensures high-quality results.

IV. Hygiene and Safety

1. Personal Hygiene Standards

Personal hygiene standards play a crucial role in nail technology practice as they contribute to ensuring a safe and hygienic environment for both the client and the technician. Maintaining high standards of personal hygiene is essential to prevent the transmission of bacteria, viruses, and other pathogens during nail reconstruction treatments.

Before commencing any treatment, it is important for the technician to ensure that all necessary precautions are taken to guarantee a clean and safe working environment. This includes thorough handwashing using warm water and antibacterial soap for at least 20 seconds to eliminate any germs present on the skin. Additionally, using alcohol-based hand sanitizers provides an additional level of sterilization.

During the treatment, it is crucial to avoid touching the face, hair, or other non-work-related objects to reduce the risk of cross-contamination between the client and the workstation. Furthermore, wearing clean, fitted clothing and keeping hair tied back and away from the face helps prevent accidental hair from falling onto tools or materials used during the treatment.

Moreover, it is important to refrain from chewing gum or eating during the treatment, as this could increase the risk of contamination of the materials and tools used. It is also advisable to avoid smoking during work, as smoke can carry germ and bacteria particles into the air, compromising the cleanliness of the work environment.

Finally, it is fundamental to adhere to personal hygiene regulations and guidelines established by relevant authorities and to stay updated regularly on best practices and latest recommendations in hygiene and safety. Investing time and effort in adopting good personal hygiene practices helps protect the health of both the client and the technician and ensures high-quality results.

2. Cleaning and Disinfection of Tools

Cleaning and disinfection of tools are crucial procedures in nail technology as they help prevent the transmission of infections from client to client and maintain a safe and hygienic work environment. It is essential to adopt accurate protocols to ensure that tools used during nail reconstruction treatments are thoroughly cleaned and sterilized.

Before using tools on a new client, a rigorous cleaning procedure is necessary to remove any dust, dirt, or previously used products. This can be done by immersing the tools in a cleaning solution and using brushes or sponges to remove unwanted particles. Special attention should be paid to hidden or hard-to-reach areas of the tools where bacteria can accumulate and proliferate.

After the initial cleaning, tools must undergo a disinfection process to completely eliminate any pathogenic microorganisms present on the tool surfaces. Disinfection can be carried out using chemical disinfectants specifically formulated for this purpose, such as alcohol-based solutions or chlorine dioxide. Tools should be fully immersed in the disinfectant solution for the time recommended by the manufacturer, ensuring effective sterilization.

Following disinfection, tools should be thoroughly dried using clean towels or low-temperature hair dryers to prevent rust formation or damage to the tools. It is important to store tools in clean, tightly sealed containers to prevent contamination by bacteria or other pathogens.

Moreover, it is essential to monitor the expiration dates of disinfectants and regularly replace disinfectant solutions to ensure effective tool sterilization. Keeping detailed records of tool cleaning and disinfection procedures is also advisable to demonstrate compliance with hygiene regulations and ensure client safety.

Investing time and effort into cleaning and disinfecting tools is indispensable for every nail technician as it helps protect client health and maintain high standards of hygiene and safety in the work environment.

3. Waste Management

Waste management is a crucial aspect of nail technology practice, as it ensures a clean, safe, and environmentally friendly work environment. During nail reconstruction treatments, various types of waste can be produced, including residues of gel, acrylic, acrygel, nail filings, and packaging materials from used products. Adopting a responsible approach to waste management is essential to reduce environmental impact and protect public health.

Before starting any treatment, it is important to have an adequate waste collection and disposal system in place that complies with local and regional regulations. This may include using separate containers for different types of waste, such as plastic, paper, and hazardous materials, as well as clearly identifying and labeling containers in accordance with current regulations.

During treatment, it is important to implement waste reduction practices, such as recycling materials whenever possible and using appropriate amounts of products to avoid excessive waste. For example, carefully measuring the amount of gel, acrylic, or acrygel used for each treatment and using only what is necessary to achieve the desired result is advisable.

After completing the treatment, proper disposal of waste in accordance with local and regional regulations is crucial. This may involve transporting waste to an authorized disposal center or coordinating with specialized waste collection services for hazardous waste management.

Furthermore, educating clients on the importance of proper waste management and encouraging them to actively participate in waste reduction and recycling efforts is important. For instance, providing information on local recycling programs and tips on reducing the environmental impact of beauty practices can be beneficial.

In conclusion, proper waste management is essential to ensure a safe, clean, and environmentally respectful work environment in nail technology. Adopting responsible waste management practices not only protects the environment but also promotes sustainability and public health.

4. Use of Personal Protective Equipment (PPE)

In the field of nail technology, the appropriate use of Personal Protective Equipment (PPE) is essential to ensure the safety of both the technician and the client during nail reconstruction treatments. PPE provides an effective barrier against potential health risks, including exposure to chemicals, toxic vapors, and bacterial contaminants. It is crucial for the technician to be well-informed about the different types of PPE available and the situations in which they should be used.

One of the most common PPE in nail technology are disposable latex or nitrile gloves. These gloves offer effective protection against liquids and chemicals used during treatments, reducing the risk of skin irritations or allergies. It is important to wear gloves throughout the entire treatment and to change them regularly to avoid cross-contamination between clients.

Additionally, respiratory masks are advisable during the application of products such as gel, acrylic, or acrygel, which can release toxic vapors during the polymerization process. Respiratory masks help protect the technician's airways from irritation and damage caused by exposure to chemical vapors, ensuring a safe and healthy working environment.

Other types of PPE that may be used during nail reconstruction treatments include protective eyewear to shield the eyes from accidental splashes of chemicals or nail filings, and disposable aprons or gowns to protect clothing from stains and contamination.

It is important for the technician to be trained in the correct use of PPE and to strictly follow safety and hygiene guidelines established by competent authorities. Adopting effective safety practices not only protects the health of the technician and the client but also promotes a professional and reliable reputation in the nail technology industry.

5. Emergency Procedures

In the field of nail technology, it is crucial to be prepared to handle any emergency situations that may arise during nail reconstruction treatments. Emergency procedures are designed to ensure the safety of the technician, the client, and anyone in the work area in the event of accidents or unexpected events. It is important to establish clear protocols and regularly practice emergency procedures to ensure a prompt and effective response when needed.

One of the primary emergency procedures involves managing chemical incidents. In case of accidental contact with irritating or corrosive chemicals, it is important to immediately flush the affected area with plenty of water and seek medical attention promptly if necessary. Technicians should be trained in identifying and managing chemicals used during treatments and know the correct handling and disposal procedures.

Another critical emergency procedure is managing cuts or wounds. In case of accidental cuts or injuries during treatments, it is essential to immediately stop bleeding by applying pressure to the wound with a clean cloth or sterile pad. Subsequently, the wound should be thoroughly cleaned with water and soap and protected with a bandage or sterile dressing to prevent infections.

It is also important to have a well-defined evacuation plan in case of emergencies such as fires or gas leaks. Staff should be trained on safe escape routes and designated assembly points to ensure orderly and safe evacuation for everyone in the work area.

Additionally, it is advisable to have a fully stocked and updated first aid kit on hand that includes all necessary items for managing common injuries. The first aid kit should be easily accessible, and staff should be trained in the correct use of the items in the kit.

Finally, conducting regular emergency drills is important to test the effectiveness of procedures and ensure that staff is adequately prepared to handle real emergency situations. Practicing emergency procedures can help reduce panic and ensure a quick and effective response when needed.

V. Nail Reconstruction with Gel: Basic Concepts

1. Introduction to Nail Reconstruction Gel

Nail reconstruction gel has become one of the most popular and versatile materials in the field of nail technology, offering a wide range of options to create long-lasting, strong, and naturally beautiful nails. This material has been developed to meet the needs of clients who desire nails that are both natural-looking and durable.

One of the distinctive features of gel is its soft and moldable consistency, which allows the technician to create custom shapes and lengths based on the client's preferences. The gel is applied in thin layers and polymerized under a UV or LED lamp, resulting in a resilient and glossy final outcome.

There are several types of gels available on the market, each with unique characteristics and properties. For instance, base gel is used as a foundational layer to enhance adhesion and prolong the longevity of the treatment, while builder gel is designed to add thickness and strength to natural nails.

The introduction to nail reconstruction gel also covers different viscosity grades of gel, which influence ease of application and the ability to sculpt nails. Thicker gels are ideal for building long and resilient nails, whereas thinner gels are used for finishing and polishing.

Throughout this chapter, we will delve into the various types of gels available on the market, their distinctive features, and best practices for application and sculpting. Practical examples and detailed instructions will be provided to enable technicians to gain comprehensive and in-depth knowledge of nail reconstruction gel.

2. Preparing the Natural Nail for Gel Application

Proper preparation of the natural nail is a crucial step in ensuring effective and long-lasting gel reconstruction. Thorough preparation not only enhances gel adhesion to the natural nail but also helps prevent issues such as lifting or premature detachment.

The first step in preparing the natural nail is removing any residual nail polish or previous nail products. It is important to ensure the nail is completely clean and free from any oil or product residue, as even the smallest contamination can compromise gel adhesion.

Next, gently push back the cuticles using a wooden cuticle stick or cuticle pusher. This step is essential to create a smooth and uniform surface for gel application, minimizing the risk of lifting or detachment.

Once the cuticles are pushed back, lightly buff the surface of the natural nail to remove the outer matte layer and promote gel adhesion. It is advisable to use a fine-grit nail file to avoid damaging the underlying nail and to achieve a smooth and even surface.

After buffing, dehydrate the nail using a specific nail dehydrator. This step helps remove any oil or moisture residue from the nail surface, further improving gel adhesion and extending the longevity of the treatment.

Finally, apply a thin layer of primer to the natural nail. Primer helps create a chemical bond between the nail and the gel, further enhancing adhesion and ensuring longer-lasting results.

Thorough preparation of the natural nail is essential for achieving optimal outcomes in gel reconstruction. Following these steps carefully will ensure a solid and long-lasting foundation for gel application, delivering a professional and resilient final result over time.

3. Gel Application: Essential Steps

The application of gel for nail reconstruction involves a series of essential steps to ensure a professional and long-lasting final result. Carefully following these steps is crucial to achieve natural-looking, resilient, and impeccable nails.

The first step in gel application is selecting the type and color of gel based on the client's preferences and desired outcome. It is important to choose a high-quality gel that is compatible with the nail type and desired final result.

Once the gel is selected, the technician must properly set up the workstation, ensuring that all necessary tools and materials are within reach and that the UV or LED lamp is turned on and ready for use.

The second step is applying the base gel on the natural nail using a precision brush to evenly distribute the gel across the nail surface. This base layer helps to enhance gel adhesion and prevent premature lifting or detachment.

After applying the base gel, the technician proceeds with building the nail using the builder gel. This thicker, self-leveling gel is applied in thin layers and precisely shaped to create the desired shape and length. It is important to work swiftly and accurately during this step to prevent the gel from drying before completing the shaping.

Once the nail is shaped, the technician cures the gel under the UV or LED lamp for the required time. During this process, it is important to carefully follow the manufacturer's instructions to ensure complete and even gel curing.

Finally, the technician refines and buffs the nail using a file and buffer to achieve a smooth and shiny surface. This final step helps perfect the overall appearance of the reconstructed nails.

Carefully following these essential steps during gel application will ensure a professional and long-lasting final result, meeting the needs and expectations of clients.

4. Gel Polymerization and Drying

Polymerization and drying of the gel are crucial phases during the nail reconstruction process. These operations ensure the solidification of the gel, guaranteeing the durability and stability of the reconstruction.

After shaping the nail with gel, it is necessary to polymerize the gel under a UV or LED lamp. This step is essential because polymerization activates the catalytic agents present in the gel, causing it to harden and solidify completely. The length of polymerization time depends on the type of gel used and the power of the lamp. It is important to carefully follow the manufacturer's instructions to ensure effective and uniform polymerization.

During the polymerization process, it is crucial to ensure that the gel is exposed to UV or LED light evenly and completely. Incomplete polymerization can cause issues such as air bubbles or the formation of sticky layers on the surface of the reconstructed nail. To avoid this, it is advisable to gently rotate the client's fingers under the lamp during the polymerization process, ensuring uniform exposure of the gel to light.

Once polymerization is complete, it is important to carefully check the solidity of the gel. Using a light touch, the technician can ensure that the gel is fully hardened and shows no flexibility or softness. If not, it is advisable to repeat the polymerization process under the lamp for the necessary time.

After polymerization, the technician can proceed with refining and polishing the reconstructed nail to achieve a flawless and professional appearance. Proper gel polymerization is essential to ensure the durability and stability of the reconstruction, providing the client with a high-quality and long-lasting final result.

5. Finishing and Polishing Reconstructed Nails with Gel

Finishing and polishing reconstructed nails with gel are crucial steps to achieve a flawless and professional final result. These operations smooth out any roughness, refine the nail shape, and give it a glossy and shiny appearance.

To begin the finishing process, it is advisable to use a fine-grit file to gently smooth the surface of the nail. This step helps to remove any irregularities or protrusions on the gel, ensuring a smooth and uniform surface. It's important to work carefully and precisely, avoiding over-filing the nail to maintain its structural integrity.

Next, a buffer can be used to further smooth the nail surface and make it even more uniform and polished. The buffer, equipped with different grains, helps to eliminate any marks left by the file and prepares the nail for the polishing phase.

Once the finishing is completed, the nail is ready for polishing to give it a shiny and glossy appearance. For this purpose, a polishing buffer or a buffing block specially designed for gel can be used. With gentle and circular movements, polish the nail surface until achieving the desired level of brightness and shine.

During the polishing phase, it's important to pay attention to the pressure applied to the buffer to avoid damaging the gel or creating scratches on the nail surface. It is recommended to work lightly and precisely, ensuring to evenly cover the entire nail surface for a consistent and professional result.

Once polishing is complete, the reconstructed nail with gel will be ready to be presented to the client, offering an impeccable and luminous appearance that meets their aesthetic expectations.

VI. Preparing the Natural Nail for Gel Reconstruction

1. Assessment of the Natural Nail Condition

Assessing the condition of the natural nail is the crucial first step in preparing for gel reconstruction. Before commencing any procedure, it is essential to thoroughly examine the nail to determine its current condition and identify any issues or anomalies.

During this assessment phase, it is important to observe several aspects of the nail, including its shape, length, thickness, and structural integrity. Any damages, breaks, or deformities present on the nail should also be examined, as they may impact the reconstruction process.

Furthermore, evaluating the condition of the cuticles and surrounding skin is essential to identify signs of inflammation, irritation, or infection. Special attention should be paid to the presence of signs of fungal or bacterial infections, which may require specific treatment before proceeding with reconstruction.

During the assessment of the natural nail, it is also advisable to discuss with the client their needs, preferences, and expectations regarding the reconstruction. This allows for customization of the treatment based on the client's specific requirements and ensures satisfactory results.

In conclusion, assessing the condition of the natural nail is a crucial step in preparing for gel reconstruction, enabling the identification of any issues and planning for a targeted and personalized intervention. A careful initial assessment contributes to ensuring the safety, effectiveness, and satisfaction of the treatment for both parties involved.

2. Removal of Nail Polish Residue and Nail Cleansing

Removing nail polish residue and cleansing the nail are two crucial steps in preparing the natural nail before gel reconstruction. This process requires meticulous care and a series of carefully executed steps to ensure a clean surface free of impurities, thereby promoting optimal gel adhesion and longevity of the reconstruction.

Firstly, it is necessary to completely remove any nail polish residue using a specific nail polish remover. This product, applied with a cotton pad, effectively removes the polish without damaging the natural nail. Attention to detail is important to ensure complete removal of color, especially along the free edge of the nail and around the cuticles.

Once the polish is removed, the nail cleansing phase begins. This process involves using a gentle cleanser or a specific nail disinfectant, which helps to remove grease, oils, and other impurities from the nail surface. This step is crucial to ensure optimal gel adhesion and prevent the formation of air bubbles or lifting during reconstruction.

After applying the cleanser or disinfectant, it is advisable to use a nail brush or wooden stick to thoroughly clean under the free edge of the nail and around the cuticles, removing any remaining polish residue or dirt. This ensures a completely clean surface prepared for gel application.

In conclusion, the removal of nail polish residue and nail cleansing are fundamental steps in preparing for gel reconstruction, ensuring a clean surface free of impurities for optimal gel application. Paying attention to these details will contribute to achieving professional and long-lasting results.

3. Cuticle Removal and Nail Bed Preparation

Cuticle removal and nail bed preparation are two essential steps in the gel nail reconstruction procedure. These processes aim to create an optimal working surface, free from obstacles and ready to receive gel evenly and durably.

To effectively and safely remove cuticles, it is advisable to use a specific cuticle solvent or soak that softens and facilitates the removal of cuticles. Alternatively, a soft cuticle gel or cream can be gently massaged onto the cuticles to further soften them. Subsequently, using a wooden stick or a specialized cuticle pusher, gently push the cuticle towards the nail bed, delicately removing any excess skin tissue. It is crucial to work with extreme gentleness to avoid trauma or injury to the surrounding skin.

After completing the cuticle removal, proceed with nail bed preparation. This step involves using a fine-grit nail drill or file to smooth out any imperfections on the surface of the natural nail and to even out the nail bed. This process not only helps to ensure a smooth and uniform surface for gel application but also improves adhesion and longevity of the reconstruction. It is important to work with delicacy and precision to avoid damaging the natural nail and to achieve optimal results.

In conclusion, cuticle removal and nail bed preparation are two critical steps in preparing the natural nail for gel reconstruction. By carefully following these procedures and working with care and precision, you can ensure a solid and long-lasting foundation for quality nail reconstruction.

4. Smoothing the Surface of the Natural Nail

Smoothing the surface of the natural nail is a crucial step in the preparation process for gel reconstruction. This procedure aims to create a uniform surface, free from irregularities and any imperfections that could compromise the adhesion and longevity of the reconstruction.

To properly smooth the nail surface, it is essential to use a high-quality file with a grit suitable for nail preparation. Opting for a medium-fine grit file is advisable as it effectively smooths the surface without damaging the natural nail.

Before starting the filing process, it's important to ensure the nail is clean and free from any remnants of polish or oils. Once confirmed, proceed with gentle and controlled movements, working evenly across the entire nail surface. It is recommended to file the nail from the free edge towards the cuticle, maintaining a constant angle to avoid damaging the nail bed.

During filing, pay attention to the lateral areas of the nail and any rough or uneven spots. These areas may require extra attention and targeted filing to ensure a completely smooth and uniform surface.

Once filing is complete, use a soft brush to remove any dust or debris to ensure a clean surface ready for gel application. This step is essential for achieving optimal results and a quality nail reconstruction.

In conclusion, smoothing the surface of the natural nail is a fundamental step in preparing for gel reconstruction. By carefully following procedures and working with care and precision, you can ensure a solid and long-lasting foundation for impeccable nail reconstruction.

5. Dehydration and Application of Primer

Dehydration and application of primer are two essential steps in preparing the natural nail before gel reconstruction. These processes prepare the nail, ensuring optimal adhesion of the gel and enhancing the longevity of the reconstruction.

Nail dehydration is a crucial step that eliminates any residues of oils, fats, or moisture from the nail surface. This process is fundamental to ensure perfect gel adhesion and to prevent premature lifting or peeling. To properly dehydrate the nail, a specific product, typically based on isopropyl alcohol, is used, which effectively removes any trace of moisture.

After dehydration, the next step is applying the primer, a chemical product designed to promote the adhesion of gel to the natural nail. The primer is carefully applied to the nail surface, avoiding contact with the surrounding skin. It's important to apply the primer only on the nail bed and prevent it from coming into contact with the cuticle or surrounding skin to avoid irritation or unwanted reactions.

Once the primer is applied, it must be allowed to dry completely before proceeding with gel application. This ensures that the primer has time to firmly adhere to the nail, creating a solid and durable base for the gel.

In conclusion, dehydration and application of primer are two crucial steps in preparing the natural nail for gel reconstruction. By carefully following procedures and working with care and precision, you can ensure a solid and long-lasting foundation for impeccable nail reconstruction.

VII. Gel Application: Essential Steps

1. Preparation of the Natural Nail

Thorough preparation of the natural nail is a fundamental step to ensure effective and long-lasting reconstruction. Before starting any gel, acrylic, or acrigel reconstruction procedure, it is essential to ensure that the natural nail is clean, healthy, and ready to receive the reconstructive material.

The first step in preparing the natural nail is to remove any nail polish residue on the nail surface. It is important to ensure that the nail is completely free of polish to guarantee optimal adhesion of the reconstructive material.

Next, proceed with the removal of cuticles and cleaning of the nail bed. Excess cuticles can interfere with the even application of gel or acrylic and compromise the durability of the treatment. Using an appropriate tool and following the proper techniques, the cuticles are gently pushed back and trimmed, leaving the nail bed clean and free of residues.

Once cuticle removal is complete, it is important to proceed with buffing the surface of the natural nail. This step helps create a slightly rough surface that promotes the adhesion of gel or acrylic. Using a fine-grit file, gently buff the nail, avoiding damage to the underlying nail bed.

Finally, before applying the primer, it is essential to dehydrate the natural nail to eliminate any residues of grease or moisture that could compromise the adhesion of the gel. This step ensures better adherence of the reconstructive material and contributes to the durability of the treatment.

In summary, preparing the natural nail is a detailed process that requires attention and precision. By following the correct steps and using the appropriate tools, you can ensure a solid foundation for high-quality nail reconstruction.

2. Application of the Primer

Applying the primer is a crucial step in preparing the natural nail before reconstruction with gel, acrylic, or acrigel. The primer is a chemical product designed to enhance the adhesion of the reconstructive material to the natural nail, ensuring longer-lasting treatment and reducing the risk of lifting or detachment.

Before applying the primer, it is important to ensure that the nail is clean and free from any residue of polish, oil, or other substances that might compromise the adhesion of the gel or acrylic. Using a specific cleanser, thoroughly clean the nail, ensuring that all residues are removed and the surface is completely dry.

Once the nail is prepared, proceed with the application of the primer. The primer is generally available in liquid form and is applied with a thin brush to the surface of the natural nail. It is important to apply the primer carefully, avoiding contact with the surrounding skin or cuticles, as it could cause irritation or allergic reactions.

After applying the primer, it is necessary to let it dry completely before proceeding with the application of gel, acrylic, or acrigel. This drying time allows the primer to form a strong and durable bond with the natural nail, ensuring optimal adhesion of the reconstructive material.

In conclusion, applying the primer is a critical step in preparing the natural nail for reconstruction. By following the correct techniques and using the primer appropriately, it is possible to ensure a solid and durable base for high-quality nail reconstruction.

3. Selection and Preparation of the Gel

The selection of the gel for nail reconstruction is a crucial step that requires careful attention and consideration. There are various types of gels available on the market, each with unique characteristics and specific uses. Before proceeding with the application, it is important to understand the differences between the various types of gels and choose the one that best suits the client's needs and the desired outcome.

Firstly, it is necessary to evaluate the gel's consistency, which can range from thick to fluid. Thicker gels are ideal for building longer and more durable nails, while more fluid gels are suitable for a thinner and more natural coverage. The choice of consistency depends on the desired effect and the preferred application technique.

Besides consistency, it is also important to consider the type of gel based on the client's needs. For example, there are single-phase gels that can be used to build the entire nail in one step, and dual-phase gels that require the application of a separate base layer and top layer. The choice between these depends on the client's personal preferences and the complexity of the work to be done.

Once the type and consistency of the gel have been selected, it is essential to prepare it correctly before application. This may include mixing the gel to ensure an even distribution of ingredients or using a specific primer to enhance the gel's adhesion to the natural nail. Additionally, it is important to ensure that the gel is at room temperature and that the tools used are clean and sterilized to prevent contamination and infection.

In conclusion, the selection and preparation of the gel are crucial steps in nail reconstruction. Understanding the characteristics of different types of gels and following the correct preparation procedures will ensure an optimal and satisfactory result for the client.

4. Gel Application Technique

The gel application technique requires precision and skill to achieve professional and long-lasting results. Before starting, make sure you have all the necessary tools and materials at hand, and prepare the workstation properly.

To begin, evaluate the client's natural nail to identify any issues or imperfections. Remove any nail polish residue and thoroughly clean the nail with a gentle cleanser to ensure good gel adhesion.

Next, prepare the nail bed by removing excess cuticles with a cutter or cuticle pusher. Be sure to work gently to avoid injuring or irritating the skin.

Once the nail is prepared, proceed to the primer application phase. Apply the primer to the surface of the natural nail, avoiding contact with the surrounding skin. The primer helps to improve the gel's adhesion to the nail, ensuring the treatment lasts longer.

At this point, you are ready to apply the gel. Use a gel brush to take a small amount of product and spread it evenly on the nail, starting from the base and moving towards the free edge. Ensure the gel is distributed evenly, avoiding clumps or product buildup.

Once the gel is applied, use a UV or LED lamp to cure the gel and set it on the nail. Follow the curing times recommended by the gel manufacturer to ensure complete drying and optimal treatment durability.

Finally, finish and polish the reconstructed gel nail to achieve a flawless result. Use a file to shape the nail and smooth out any imperfections. Apply a top coat to protect the gel and give a shiny, glossy effect.

By carefully following these steps and practicing consistently, you will be able to master the gel application technique and offer high-quality treatments to your clients.

5. Drying and Curing

After applying the gel to the nail, it is crucial to ensure proper drying and curing to guarantee the longevity and durability of the treatment. This process is essential to securely set the gel on the nail and prevent potential damage or premature lifting.

First, make sure to use a high-quality UV or LED lamp capable of providing effective and even curing of the gel. Before starting the drying process, check that the lamp is in perfect working condition and that the curing times are correctly set according to the gel manufacturer's instructions.

Once the nail is positioned inside the lamp, initiate the drying and curing cycle and carefully follow the recommended times. During this process, it is important that the gel is exposed to UV or LED light for the required time to ensure complete catalyzation and hardening of the material.

During curing, pay particular attention to avoiding sudden movements or temperature changes, as these could compromise the final result. Keep the nail inside the lamp for the entire duration of the drying cycle, ensuring that every part of the gel is evenly exposed to the light.

Once curing is complete, check that the gel is fully hardened by gently touching it with a finger. If the gel feels soft or sticky, repeat the drying process for additional time until a solid and durable consistency is achieved.

Finally, remove any residual tackiness with a cotton pad soaked in cleanser, and proceed with the finishing and polishing phase of the reconstructed nail. By carefully following these steps, you will be able to achieve professional and long-lasting results in gel nail reconstruction.

6. Finishing and Polishing

After completing the gel curing process, it's essential to focus on the finishing and polishing stages to achieve a flawless and professional final result. This phase smooths out any irregularities on the reconstructed nail surface, ensuring an even and glossy finish.

To start the finishing process, use a fine-grit buffer to gently smooth the gel surface. Move the buffer in gentle, circular motions, being careful not to apply too much pressure to avoid damaging the nail structure. This step is crucial for eliminating any roughness, small bumps, or excess gel residues.

After smoothing the surface, apply a clear top coat polish to protect the gel and enhance the shine of the reconstructed nail. Make sure to apply the polish in a thin, even layer, avoiding excess that could compromise the treatment's longevity.

Once the top coat is applied, proceed with the polishing stage to achieve a bright, professional finish. Use a polishing buffer or a shining file to gently buff the polish surface, giving the reconstructed nail a glossy and shiny finish.

During polishing, pay special attention to maintaining a consistent and even motion, avoiding excessive pressure on the nail surface. This final step is crucial for achieving a perfect, long-lasting finish that highlights the gel reconstruction work.

Finally, complete the finishing and polishing process by applying a nourishing cuticle oil around the nail edges, hydrating and strengthening the surrounding skin. This will help maintain the health and beauty of the reconstructed nails over time, ensuring long-lasting and satisfying results.

VIII. Advanced Techniques for Gel Reconstruction

1. Using Tips and Forms for Nail Reconstruction

The use of tips and forms in nail reconstruction is a fundamental practice for professional nail artists. Tips, which can be made of plastic or resin, are prefabricated extensions applied to the end of the natural nail to create additional length. Forms, on the other hand, are adhesive paper or plastic sheets that are molded around the end of the nail to create a customized shape before applying gel or acrylic.

Using tips offers a quick solution for nail lengthening, allowing nail artists to create uniform and consistent lengths without relying on the client's natural nail length. This method is particularly useful for clients with short or damaged nails who desire a longer, more elegant appearance.

Conversely, using forms allows for greater customization, enabling nail artists to shape the nails according to the client's preferences and specific nail anatomy. Forms also offer more flexibility in creating various nail shapes, such as coffin tips or almond-shaped nails.

Regardless of the chosen method, both tips and forms require accurate practice and in-depth knowledge of application techniques to ensure high-quality results. Nail artists must be able to select the correct size and shape of tips and position them correctly on the natural nail. Similarly, they must be skilled in shaping the forms to achieve a smooth and even surface before applying the gel or acrylic.

Additionally, it is essential for nail artists to understand how to remove tips and forms properly without damaging the underlying natural nail. Improper removal can lead to damage to the natural nail, compromising the overall health and integrity of the client's nails.

In conclusion, using tips and forms is a key practice in gel or acrylic nail reconstruction. With the right knowledge and practice, nail artists can effectively use these tools to create stunning results and meet their clients' aesthetic needs.

2. Gel Extension Techniques: Dual Form and Reverse Technique

Gel extension techniques provide nail artists with a wide range of options to create long and perfectly shaped nails. Two of the most popular techniques are the use of Dual Forms and the Reverse Technique.

Dual Forms are innovative tools that allow nail artists to easily create nails with a uniform shape and precise length. These forms come pre-formed with a natural curve and a free edge, making them ideal for creating pointed, almond-shaped, or square nails. To use Dual Forms, the artist applies gel onto the form and places it onto the natural nail, shaping and leveling the gel according to the desired form. Once the gel is cured under a UV or LED lamp, the Dual Form can be removed to reveal perfectly sculpted nails ready for finishing.

The Reverse Technique is another advanced method that enables nail artists to create long and thin nails with a natural appearance. In this technique, instead of applying gel to the nail tip, the artist spreads the gel on the underside of the natural nail, near the nail bed. Using a thin and precise brush, the gel is molded and pushed towards the nail tip, creating a gradual lengthening and natural shape. Once the desired length is achieved, the gel is cured under a UV or LED lamp and refined to achieve a flawless look.

Both of these techniques require practice and skill to execute successfully, but once mastered, they offer stunning and long-lasting results. Nail artists should experiment with both techniques to determine which best suits their preferences and meets their clients' needs.

Moreover, it is important for nail artists to understand the precautions to take during gel application and when using different techniques. Proper preparation of the natural nail, the use of high-quality products, and attention to detail are crucial for achieving optimal results and ensuring client satisfaction.

In conclusion, gel extension techniques such as Dual Forms and the Reverse Technique provide nail artists with a range of options to create long and perfectly shaped nails. With practice and proper knowledge, stunning results can be achieved to meet the aesthetic demands of even the most discerning clients.

3. Gel Reconstruction on Soft or Damaged Nails

Reconstructing nails with gel on soft or damaged nails requires particular attention and a targeted approach to ensure optimal and lasting results. Soft nails can result from various factors such as moisture and water absorption, excessive use of chemicals, or conditions like onycholysis. Additionally, damaged nails may exhibit cracks, chips, or surface irregularities, making reconstruction a delicate yet essential operation to restore the appearance and health of the nails.

Effectively addressing gel reconstruction on soft or damaged nails involves following a series of key steps. Firstly, it's crucial to carefully assess the condition of the nails to identify any issues or conditions that may affect the reconstruction process. This assessment should include a visual examination of the nails as well as a discussion with the client to understand the nail history and any previous health issues or treatments received.

Once the nail conditions have been evaluated, thorough preparation of the nail surface for gel application is essential. This may involve gently removing nail polish residue, cleaning the nail, and pushing back cuticles. Additionally, lightly buffing the nail surface may be necessary to smooth out any irregularities or protrusions that could interfere with the even application of the gel.

After preparing the nail, selecting the most suitable gel for the client's needs and the nail condition is fundamental. There are various types of gels available, each with unique characteristics and properties. For instance, builder gels are ideal for reinforcing weak or damaged nails, while finishing gels offer a glossy and long-lasting finish.

Once the appropriate gel has been chosen, it's essential to apply it with precision and care, ensuring to evenly cover the entire nail surface and sculpt the gel according to the desired shape. During application, it's important to avoid excess gel and work in thin layers to ensure better adhesion and a more natural finish.

Finally, proper curing of the gel under a UV or LED lamp is essential to ensure complete polymerization and optimal product durability. After curing, you can proceed with the refinement and polishing of the nails to achieve an impeccable result that meets the client's aesthetic needs.

4. Creating Special Effects and Decorations with Gel

Creating special effects and decorations with gel offers a wide range of creative possibilities to enhance nail reconstructions. Among the most popular techniques is using colors, glitter, rhinestones, and other decorative elements to add style and personality to reconstructed nails.

To begin with, it's important to have a variety of colored gels and glitters of different types and sizes on hand to experiment with various combinations and styles. Before applying decorative gel, ensure that the base layer has been fully cured and that the nail surface has been properly prepared.

One of the most common techniques for creating special effects is incorporating glitter directly into clear or colored gel to achieve a bright and sparkling effect. Thin brushes can also be used to draw patterns or create gradients using multiple colors of gel.

Additionally, applying rhinestones and beads can add a touch of elegance and glamour to nails. These elements can be placed on nails using an orange stick or nail art tweezers and then secured with a layer of clear gel.

It's important to exercise precision and attention to detail during the decoration process to achieve clean and professional results. Regular practice and experimenting with different techniques will help improve skills and develop a unique and distinctive style.

Finally, after completing the decoration, be sure to seal everything with a layer of top coat gel to ensure long-lasting durability and a glossy, finished appearance.

5. Gel Application on C-Curve and Tunnel-Shaped Nails

Applying gel on nails with pronounced C-curves or tunnels requires particular attention and skill to ensure uniform and long-lasting reconstruction. Nails with C-curves or tunnels can pose additional challenges during the gel application process, but with the right techniques, excellent results can be achieved.

To begin with, it's important to carefully assess the shape and structure of the natural nail before starting the reconstruction. Nails with C-curves or tunnels may require additional preparation to level the surface and create a smooth base for gel application.

During nail preparation, use a file to smooth out any irregularities and create a smooth, even surface. It's important to remove any bumps or ridges to prevent gel buildup and unwanted thickness.

Next, select the appropriate gel for the nail type and specific curve. Thicker gels can be used to fill tunnels and create a more uniform surface, while more fluid gels are ideal for adapting to the nail's natural curves.

During gel application, work with fluid and precise movements to evenly distribute the product along the entire nail surface. It's important to work in thin layers and add gel only where necessary to avoid excessive buildup that could compromise the longevity and strength of the reconstruction.

Once the gel is applied, you can further shape and define the form using a gel brush and monomer or isopropyl liquid to smooth and level the surface. Ensure to work with precision and attention to detail to achieve impeccable shape and an even surface.

Finally, cure the gel thoroughly using a UV or LED lamp to ensure complete polymerization and optimal durability of the reconstruction. Verify that the gel is fully hardened before proceeding with nail finishing and polishing.

In conclusion, applying gel on C-curve and tunnel-shaped nails requires a combination of skills, attention to detail, and proper preparation to achieve professional and long-lasting results. With practice and mastery of appropriate techniques, high-quality reconstructions can be created on any type of nail.

6. Safe and Proper Removal of Gel

Safe and proper removal of gel is a crucial step to ensure the health and integrity of natural nails after reconstruction. Improper or aggressive removal can damage the nail plate and lead to weakening or breakage of the nails. Here are some tips and techniques for safely and effectively removing gel:

Firstly, it's important to use tools and products specifically designed for gel removal, such as dedicated gel removers or nail wraps. Avoid using metallic or abrasive tools that could damage the nail surface.

Before starting removal, prepare the work area and protect surrounding skin with cuticle oil or moisturizing cream to prevent irritation or dryness.

To remove the gel, saturate a cotton pad with gel remover and wrap it around the nail. Use nail wraps or aluminum foil to secure the cotton pad and ensure even application of the remover.

Allow the remover to sit for a few minutes to soften the gel and facilitate its removal. Avoid forcing or pulling the gel, as this could damage the natural nail.

After allowing the remover to work, remove the cotton pad and use a cuticle pusher or wooden tool to gently lift the gel from the nail surface. If the gel doesn't come off easily, repeat the soaking process with the remover and let it sit a bit longer.

Once all the gel is removed, use a soft file to smooth out any remaining residue or imperfections on the nail surface. Avoid over-filing to prevent damage to the upper layer of the nail.

Finally, moisturize and nourish the nails and cuticles with cuticle oil or moisturizing cream to restore hydration and flexibility after gel removal.

Remember, gentle and accurate gel removal is essential for maintaining the health and beauty of natural nails. With proper technique and attention to detail, gel can be removed safely and effectively, preparing nails for subsequent reconstruction or maintenance.

7. Troubleshooting Common Issues during Gel Reconstruction

During gel reconstruction, various common issues may arise that require prompt and accurate solutions to ensure optimal results. Here are some of the most frequent problems and their respective solutions:

Air Bubbles Formation: Air bubbles can form during gel application, compromising the final appearance and longevity of the reconstruction. To prevent this issue, it is crucial to apply the gel in thin, even layers, avoiding trapping air between the gel and the natural nail. Additionally, using a specialized tool such as a brush or cuticle pusher to push out any air bubbles during application can be helpful.

Peeling or Lifting of Gel: If the gel peels or lifts from the edges of the nail, it may be due to poor adhesion or incorrect application. To resolve this problem, ensure thorough preparation of the natural nail by completely removing moisture and cuticles. Apply the gel in thin layers and seal the nail edges well to prevent lifting.

Crowning or C-Curve Formation: In some cases, the gel may tend to form unwanted crowns or C-curves on the nail. To correct this situation, it is important to carefully file the nail surface during reconstruction, ensuring to maintain a natural and uniform shape. Additionally, using specific modeling techniques, such as applying gel on C-curves, can correct any irregularities.

Dull or Uneven Result: If the gel appears dull or exhibits irregularities on the surface, it may require more precise finishing or the use of higher-quality gel. Ensure to apply the gel evenly and cure it properly under a UV or LED lamp to achieve a smooth and glossy surface. Additionally, using finishing products like top coat or polishing gel can enhance the brightness and durability of the final result.

Successfully addressing these common issues during gel reconstruction requires practice, attention to detail, and knowledge of correct techniques. With experience and dedication, achieving professional and satisfying results is possible, ensuring the beauty and health of your clients' nails.

IX. Finishing and Polishing Gel Reconstructed Nails

1. Preliminary Procedures for Finishing

Preliminary procedures for finishing represent a crucial phase in the gel nail reconstruction process. This step is essential to ensure a high-quality and long-lasting final result. Before beginning the finishing phase, it is vital to ensure that the gel application has been performed correctly and that the reconstructed nail is solid and well-adhered to the natural nail.

The first step involves carefully examining each reconstructed nail to identify any irregularities or defects in the gel application. This visual inspection is fundamental for spotting any air bubbles, protrusions, or imperfections on the nail surface that could compromise the quality of the final work.

Next, it is advisable to perform a light filing of the reconstructed nail surface to smooth out any protrusions and achieve a smooth and even surface. This operation can be done using fine-grit files or buffers specifically designed for gel. It is important to be cautious during this phase to avoid removing too much material and compromising the thickness of the reconstructed nail.

Once the preliminary filing is completed, the nails should be thoroughly cleaned using a specific cleanser or degreasing product. This step is essential to remove any gel residue, dust, or oils from the nail surface and adequately prepare the base for the application of the top coat and polishing phase.

Finally, it is recommended to carefully check the adhesion of the gel to the natural nail and ensure that there are no detachments or lifting along the free edge of the nail. If necessary, small corrections or repairs can be made using the appropriate gel and a LED or UV lamp for curing.

In summary, the preliminary procedures for finishing are fundamental to ensure a high-quality final result and guarantee the durability and strength of the gel reconstruction. Paying attention to details and performing each step with care and precision will contribute to achieving a professional and flawless job.

2. Gel Filing Techniques

Gel filing techniques are a crucial aspect of the finishing phase for reconstructed nails. Proper filing not only ensures an impeccable aesthetic result but also helps improve gel adhesion, reconstruction durability, and client comfort. Various techniques and tools can be employed to achieve effective and precise filing.

Firstly, it is important to choose the right grit of the file according to the specific needs of the job. For removing large amounts of material or correcting significant irregularities, a coarser grit file is recommended, while finer grit is preferred for finishing and detail work. Filing can be done manually using hand files of different shapes and sizes, or with the help of electric tools such as e-files or sanders.

During filing, it is important to maintain a smooth and controlled motion to avoid damaging the natural nail or nail bed. It is advisable to work with light pressure and gentle movements, avoiding excessive force that could damage the gel layer and cause thin fractures or cracks.

Once the initial filing is completed to smooth the nail surface and remove any imperfections, you can proceed with detailing. This phase requires particular attention to the nail contours and the desired shape, which can be achieved using horseshoe-shaped files, buffers, or other specific tools.

Throughout the filing process, it is important to regularly check the result and correct any mistakes or asymmetries to ensure a uniform and harmonious final outcome. It is advisable to work patiently and precisely, paying attention to details and aiming for a balance between the shape, length, and thickness of the reconstructed nail.

Finally, once filing is complete, it is recommended to thoroughly clean the nails to remove any dust or gel residue and prepare them for the polishing phase.

3. Using Buffers and Files for Finishing

Using buffers and files during the finishing phase is essential for achieving a flawless final result on gel-reconstructed nails. These tools are designed to smooth, polish, and define the nail surface, ensuring a smooth, shiny, and uniform finish.

Buffers are double-sided devices that feature different grits on each side. These tools allow you to smooth the nail surface, eliminating any irregularities, imperfections, or dullness. The finer grit of the buffer is used to polish the nail, giving it a shiny and smooth appearance. When using a buffer, it is important to apply light pressure and work with gentle, circular motions to avoid damaging the nail surface or the gel.

Files are essential tools for detailing and defining the shape of the nail. There are various types of files, including horseshoe files, almond files, square files, and pointed files. Each type of file is designed to fit different nail shapes and personal preferences of the client.

When using files, it is important to follow the natural shape of the nail and maintain a symmetrical and harmonious profile. Files can be used to correct any asymmetries, perfect the contours, and adjust the length of the nail according to the client's preferences.

Once the filing with files is complete, you can proceed to the final buffing using the buffer to smooth and polish the nail. This additional step helps achieve an ultra-smooth and shiny finish, enhancing the overall appearance of the gel reconstruction.

In conclusion, using buffers and files during the finishing phase is crucial to ensure a professional and high-quality result in gel nail reconstruction. These tools allow for a uniform, smooth, and shiny surface, meeting the aesthetic and style needs of the client.

4. Applying the Top Coat

Applying the top coat is one of the final crucial steps in finishing gel-reconstructed nails. This final layer not only gives the nail a glossy and shiny appearance but also provides additional protection to the underlying gel, extending its durability and resistance.

Before applying the top coat, it is important to ensure that the nail surface is completely smoothed and free of any gel or dust residues. This preliminary step ensures that the top coat adheres evenly and dries without irregularities.

The top coat can be applied in a thin, even layer using a specific gel brush or a sponge applicator. During application, it is essential to avoid excess product that could cause drips or air bubbles.

Once the top coat is applied, the nail must be cured under a UV or LED lamp to ensure complete drying and hardening of the gel. This curing process can take 30 to 60 seconds, depending on the type of lamp used and the brand of the top coat.

After curing, it is advisable to carefully check the nail for any irregularities or imperfections and correct them if necessary. Any excess top coat can be gently removed using a cotton ball soaked in a specific gel solvent, ensuring a flawless finish.

Once the top coat application and curing are complete, the nail will be shiny, glossy, and protected. The top coat enhances the overall appearance of the gel reconstruction, giving the nails a professional and long-lasting finish.

5. Polishing Techniques

Polishing techniques represent the final step in achieving a flawless finish for gel-reconstructed nails. This process not only adds an extra level of shine to the nail surface but also helps make the reconstruction more resilient and long-lasting.

Before beginning the polishing process, it is essential to ensure that the nail is completely dry and cured after the application of the top coat. Any residue of uncured product could compromise the final polishing result.

To achieve a perfectly shiny surface, various techniques and tools can be used. Among the most common are buffers and polishing pads, designed to eliminate any surface imperfections and make the nail uniformly glossy.

During the polishing process, it is important to work gently and precisely to avoid damaging the underlying gel or causing scratches on the nail surface. It is recommended to use light, circular motions, gradually moving from one side of the nail to the other to ensure even polishing.

In addition to traditional buffers and polishing pads, there are also more advanced tools and accessories, such as polishing files and four-sided polishing blocks, which allow for even more precise and brilliant results.

Once the polishing is complete, it is advisable to carefully check the nail for any imperfections or irregularities and correct them if necessary. Any signs of dullness or scratches can be removed using additional polishing steps or light localized corrections.

Polishing gel-reconstructed nails is thus a crucial step to ensure a flawless and professional final result. With the right techniques and appropriate tools, it is possible to achieve a shiny and glossy effect that enhances the beauty of the hands to the fullest.

6. Tips for a Perfect Finish

To achieve a perfect finish on gel-reconstructed nails, it is essential to follow some practical tips that ensure a professional and long-lasting result.

Firstly, pay close attention to the preparation of the natural nail before applying the gel. This includes the proper removal of nail polish residue, cleaning the nail, and removing excess cuticles. A well-prepared base ensures better gel adhesion and a uniform surface to work on.

During the gel application, it is advisable to use moderate amounts of product and distribute it evenly on the nail. Avoid excess gel that could cause excessive thickness or irregularities in the reconstruction.

During the gel curing phase, make sure to carefully follow the manufacturer's instructions and use a high-quality UV or LED lamp to ensure complete and even curing of the product.

When filing and finishing, use high-quality tools and work gently to avoid damaging the natural nail or the reconstruction. Maintain a uniform and harmonious shape, avoiding sharp edges or surface irregularities on the nail.

During polishing, use good quality buffers and polishing pads, and work with light, circular motions to achieve a shiny and uniform finish.

Finally, after the complete finishing, apply a high-quality top coat to protect the reconstruction and prolong its durability. Ensure that the edges of the nail are well sealed to prevent the gel from lifting.

By following these tips and using the appropriate techniques, it is possible to achieve a perfect finish on gel-reconstructed nails, ensuring professional and satisfying results for the client.

X. Troubleshooting and Solving Common Problems in Gel Reconstruction

1. Addressing Lifting: Tips for Long-Lasting Gel Adhesion

Gel lifting from nails can be one of the most frustrating issues for both nail technicians and clients. However, several strategies can be adopted to ensure long-lasting gel adhesion and prevent premature lifting.

First and foremost, it is crucial to thoroughly prepare the natural nail before applying the gel. This includes completely removing moisture and oil from the nail surface using specific prep products like primers and dehydrators. Additionally, ensuring that the nail is completely dry before proceeding with the gel application is essential for good adhesion.

Another important consideration is the proper preparation of the nail surface. Using buffers and files to remove any cuticle residue and gently smooth the nail surface can promote better gel adhesion. It's also important to pay attention to the shape of the nail, ensuring it is uniform and free of irregularities that could compromise the gel's hold.

During the gel application, make sure to properly seal the edges of the nail to prevent premature lifting. Apply a thin, even layer of gel over the entire nail surface, ensuring complete coverage without creating excessive thickness.

Finally, it is important to educate the client on the importance of maintenance and appropriate behaviors to preserve the gel's adhesion. This can include advice on avoiding using nails as tools and exposure to abrasive chemicals that could compromise the gel's hold.

By carefully following these tips and adopting correct application techniques, it is possible to achieve long-lasting gel adhesion and ensure client satisfaction.

2. Troublesome Bubbles: How to Avoid and Fix Their Formation

Air bubbles are one of the most common issues during gel nail reconstruction, and they can be both annoying and unsightly. To effectively avoid and resolve them, it's essential to understand the underlying causes of their formation and adopt the right precautions during the gel application process.

Air bubbles can form for several reasons, including overly quick application of the gel, using subpar or low-quality products, humidity in the work environment, or applying the gel too thickly. Therefore, it's crucial to take various measures to prevent their formation.

First, ensure you work in a well-ventilated environment with minimal humidity, as moisture can trap air bubbles under the gel during the curing process. Use high-quality products and closely follow the manufacturer's instructions to ensure proper gel application.

During gel application, avoid abrupt and overly rapid movements that could create air bubbles. Use a slow and precise technique to evenly distribute the gel on the nail, avoiding excessive layering and thickness.

If, despite these precautions, air bubbles still occur during gel application, they can be corrected promptly. Use a gel brush to gently break the air bubbles on the nail surface before the gel is fully cured. Then, you can add a thin layer of gel to fill any gaps and smooth the nail surface again to ensure an even finish.

By carefully following these tips and adopting the correct application techniques, you can effectively prevent the formation of air bubbles and achieve professional and flawless results in gel nail reconstruction.

3. Gel Stubborn: Solutions for Perfect Polymerization

When facing issues with gel polymerization, also known as "gel stubbornness," it can be frustrating and discouraging. However, there are several solutions and strategies that can help ensure perfect gel polymerization and achieve satisfactory results.

Firstly, it's important to carefully follow the manufacturer's instructions regarding the timing and method of gel polymerization. Use a high-quality UV or LED lamp and ensure it is properly calibrated to ensure uniform and complete polymerization of the gel on all nails.

If the gel appears not to polymerize properly, it may be helpful to closely examine the gel application process. Ensure to apply a thin and even layer of gel on each nail and avoid excessive overlapping of layers, as too much gel thickness can hinder the polymerization process.

Additionally, check that the gel is not expired and has been stored properly. Expired or improperly stored gels may present polymerization issues. If necessary, replace the gel with a fresh and high-quality product to ensure optimal results.

If despite these precautions the problem persists, it is advisable to contact the gel supplier for specific assistance and advice. Corrections in gel application technique or a more thorough analysis of working conditions may be needed to resolve the polymerization issue.

In summary, addressing the issue of gel stubbornness requires patience, attention to detail, and a proper understanding of gel application technique. By following the right precautions and adopting appropriate solutions, it is possible to achieve perfect gel polymerization and professional results in nail reconstruction.

4. Resistance to Retraction: Strategies for Intact and Long-lasting Gel

When it comes to ensuring resistance to gel retraction and maintaining durable reconstructed nails over time, adopting various strategies and precautions during the application and care process is crucial.

Firstly, it's important to ensure thorough preparation of the natural nail before applying the gel. Completely remove any nail polish residue and clean the nail thoroughly to ensure a clean, oil-free surface. Additionally, gently buff the nail surface to promote optimal gel adhesion.

Proper application of primer is essential to enhance gel adhesion to the natural nail and minimize the risk of retraction. Apply the primer evenly and avoid excess product to prevent retraction or lifting of the gel.

During gel application, ensure to work in thin, even layers to ensure even distribution of the product and better adhesion to the natural nail. Avoid excess gel on the nail edges and properly seal the edges to prevent gel retraction and lifting.

After gel polymerization, it's important to complete the process with careful finishing and polishing of the nails. Use high-quality buffers and files to gently smooth the gel surface and remove any imperfections. Apply a finishing top coat to protect the gel and extend the longevity of the reconstruction.

Finally, educating clients on the importance of daily care for reconstructed nails can help maintain gel integrity over time. Recommend cuticle oils and moisturizing creams to keep nails and surrounding skin healthy and prevent premature gel retraction.

By following these strategies and best practices, it is possible to ensure reconstructed nails with gel that are resistant to retraction and long-lasting, providing professional and satisfying results to clients.

5. Thinner is Better: Techniques to Avoid Excessive Thickness

To achieve optimal results in gel nail reconstruction, it's essential to adopt targeted techniques to avoid excessive product thickness, ensuring a natural appearance and prolonged durability of the reconstruction.

Firstly, during gel application, it's important to work with thin, even layers. Applying too much gel in one layer can lead to excessive thickness and compromise the natural look of the reconstructed nail. Use an appropriately sized brush and evenly distribute the gel across the entire nail surface, avoiding product buildup.

Furthermore, paying particular attention to the nail edges during gel application is crucial. Avoid overloading the edges with product and ensure they are properly sealed to prevent excessive thickness and gel lifting.

During the nail shaping and gel building phase, it's advisable to use layering techniques to gradually add volume and shape, avoiding the creation of unwanted thickness. Work patiently and precisely to sculpt the gel nail gently and in a controlled manner, adding only what's necessary to achieve the desired shape.

To ensure a smooth and even surface, it's important to gently buff and file the gel after polymerization. Use high-quality buffers and files to remove any irregularities and refine the nail shape without compromising its structural integrity.

Lastly, educating clients on the importance of maintaining a proper maintenance routine can help prevent excessive thickness in gel reconstruction. Recommend cuticle oils and moisturizing creams to keep nails and surrounding skin healthy, minimizing the risk of product buildup and gel lifting.

By following these techniques and recommended practices, it's possible to avoid excessive thickness in gel nail reconstruction, ensuring professional and long-lasting results over time.

6. Protected Skin: Preventing and Managing Unwanted Skin Reactions

Protecting the skin during the gel nail reconstruction process is crucial to prevent and manage any unwanted skin reactions. Before starting the procedure, it's important to instruct the client on the importance of keeping the skin around the nails hydrated and protected.

To avoid potential skin irritations during gel application, it's advisable to use products specifically formulated to protect sensitive skin. Applying a moisturizing cream or protective lotion to the skin surrounding the nails before starting the procedure can help create a protective barrier, reducing the risk of contact irritations from the gel.

During the preparation of the natural nail, it's essential to pay particular attention to handling tools and chemicals. Using protective gloves during filing and buffing can help shield the skin from potentially irritating substances present in the gel and other products used during the procedure.

Furthermore, it's advisable to avoid direct contact of the gel with the surrounding skin during application. Using a specialized spatula to apply the gel on the nail and preventing the product from touching the skin can help reduce the risk of skin irritations.

If unwanted skin reactions occur during or after the gel nail reconstruction procedure, it's important to act promptly to manage the issue. Gently removing the gel from the affected skin using a cotton pad soaked in gel remover can help reduce irritation and prevent any complications.

Lastly, educating the client on the importance of following a proper skincare routine can help prevent future unwanted skin reactions. Recommending the use of moisturizing creams and cuticle oils enriched with soothing and nourishing ingredients can help maintain healthy and protected skin, minimizing the risk of skin irritations during and after the gel nail reconstruction procedure.

By following these precautions and recommended practices, it's possible to protect the skin during the gel nail reconstruction procedure and prevent any unwanted skin reactions, ensuring a safe and comfortable experience for the client.

7. Secure Adhesion: Tips for Reliable Attachment

To ensure a secure and long-lasting adhesion of the gel during nail reconstruction, it's essential to follow a series of tips and recommended practices.

Before starting the procedure, ensure that the natural nail is properly prepared and cleaned. Completely remove any nail polish residue and thoroughly cleanse the nail with a specific cleanser to ensure a clean surface free from oils or residues that could compromise the gel adhesion.

Next, use a high-quality primer to prepare the nail and enhance the gel adhesion. Apply the primer evenly over the entire nail surface and allow it to dry completely before proceeding with gel application.

During gel application, ensure to distribute the product evenly without creating excessive thickness. Use a high-quality brush to apply the gel in thin, uniform layers, avoiding contact with the surrounding skin and cuticles.

Furthermore, pay attention to the proper gel polymerization using a high-quality UV or LED lamp. Follow the manufacturer's instructions and expose the nail to light for the required time to ensure complete polymerization and a secure bond of the gel.

During the polymerization phase, it's important to monitor the process carefully and ensure that the gel is properly cured before proceeding with the next stages of nail reconstruction. If necessary, expose the nail to light for additional time to ensure complete polymerization and enhanced gel adhesion.

Finally, recommend to the client to follow a proper nail care routine to maintain the gel in optimal condition and ensure secure adhesion over time. Suggest the use of cuticle oils and moisturizing creams to keep nails and surrounding skin soft and hydrated, thereby extending the longevity of the gel and ensuring a secure, long-lasting hold.

By following these tips and recommended practices, it's possible to ensure a secure and long-lasting adhesion of the gel during nail reconstruction, providing the client with satisfying and durable results.

8. Sustaining Brilliance: Maintaining Transparent and Glossy Gel

To maintain the transparency and glossy appearance of gel over time, it's important to follow a series of practices and precautions that preserve the original look of reconstructed nails. Initially, it's crucial to use high-quality products, including transparent gels and top coats, which feature a resilient and durable formula.

During gel application, ensure to distribute it evenly without creating excessive thickness to avoid the formation of air bubbles or irregularities that could compromise the transparency and glossiness of the gel. Use a good-quality brush and apply the gel in thin layers, polymerizing each layer carefully to ensure optimal adhesion and a smooth, uniform surface.

After complete gel polymerization, it's advisable to perform meticulous finishing using specially designed files and buffers to smooth the surface and remove any imperfections. Avoid over-filing the surface, as it could dull the gel's brilliance and make the surface appear matte.

Next, apply a layer of high-quality transparent top coat to protect the gel and impart a glossy, shiny finish. Ensure to apply the top coat evenly without creating air bubbles, polymerizing the product carefully to achieve a smooth and shiny surface.

To sustain the transparency and brilliance of the gel over time, it's advisable to advise the client to follow a proper nail care routine, avoiding exposure to harsh chemicals and protecting hands during daily activities. Recommend the use of cuticle oils and moisturizing creams to keep nails and surrounding skin hydrated and soft, thus helping to preserve the gel's brilliance and extend its longevity.

By following these practices and recommendations, it's possible to ensure that the gel remains transparent and glossy over time, offering clients impeccably reconstructed nails that are long-lasting and visually appealing.

9. Natural Radiance: Avoiding Unwanted Whitening

To maintain the natural radiance of nails reconstructed with gel and avoid unwanted whitening, it's essential to take precautions during application and nail care. First and foremost, using high-quality transparent gels without whitening or dulling agents is crucial to preserve the natural look of nails.

During gel application, avoid excess product and ensure even distribution over the entire nail surface. Pay particular attention to cuticles and nail edges, where gel can accumulate and cause unwanted whitening. Use a good-quality brush and work with precision to achieve uniform and transparent coverage.

After gel polymerization, perform careful finishing using gentle files and buffers to smooth the surface and remove any irregularities. Avoid over-filing the nail surface, as this could compromise the brilliance and transparency of the gel.

Furthermore, it's advisable to avoid exposure to harsh chemicals that could cause whitening or dullness of the gel. Recommend that the client wear protective gloves during household chores or work involving the use of aggressive detergents or solvents.

To maintain the natural radiance of nails reconstructed with gel, educate the client about the importance of a proper nail care routine, including daily moisturization and the application of cuticle oils to keep nails and surrounding skin soft and hydrated.

Lastly, advise the client to avoid damaging habits such as nail biting or using nails as tools, as these can damage the gel and compromise its natural radiance over time.

By following these precautions and recommendations, it's possible to avoid unwanted whitening and preserve the natural radiance of nails reconstructed with gel, providing clients with impeccable and long-lasting results.

10. Handling Lifted Sides: Strategies for Long-Lasting Reconstruction

To address lifted sides during gel reconstruction and ensure optimal durability, it's essential to adopt various preventive and corrective strategies. Firstly, during the preparation of the natural nail, ensure complete removal of cuticle residue and gently buff the nail surface to promote optimal gel adhesion.

During gel application, pay particular attention to the nail edges and ensure proper sealing along the sides to prevent premature lifting. Use specialized tools like a fine brush or wooden stick to evenly distribute the gel along the nail edges, avoiding excess product that could cause lifting.

Moreover, using high-quality gel with strong adhesion and low tendency to shrinkage is advisable to ensure optimal reconstruction durability. During gel polymerization, carefully follow the manufacturer's instructions and use high-quality UV or LED lamps to achieve complete and uniform gel curing across the entire nail surface.

If lifting occurs during or after gel application, gently use a fine-grit file to level the nail surface and remove any irregularities. Subsequently, apply a thin layer of finishing gel to seal the work and enhance the longevity of the reconstruction.

Educating the client on the importance of proper nail maintenance, avoiding using nails as tools, and protecting them during strenuous manual activities can help prevent lifting and prolong the reconstruction's durability.

By implementing these preventive and corrective strategies, it's possible to successfully manage lifted sides during gel reconstruction and ensure long-lasting, impeccable results.

XI. Nail Reconstruction with Acrylic: Basic Concepts

1. Preparing the Natural Nail for Acrylic Reconstruction

Proper preparation of the natural nail is a crucial step to ensure a quality acrylic reconstruction and long-lasting adherence. Before starting the procedure, it's essential to perform several operations to make sure the nail is optimally ready to receive the acrylic material.

The first step involves thoroughly cleaning the nail and surrounding areas using a gentle cleanser to remove any residual oils, lotions, or previously applied nail polish. This allows the acrylic material to firmly adhere to the natural nail, reducing the risk of premature lifting.

Next, it is vital to remove the superficial layer of the nail using a soft file or buffer to eliminate any dead skin cells and create a rougher surface, which helps promote the adhesion of the acrylic product.

Once the nail surface preparation is complete, it is important to take care of the cuticles by gently pushing them back towards the nail bed using a cuticle pusher and, if necessary, removing any excess cuticles with appropriate tweezers or cuticle trimmers. This step not only improves the aesthetic of the nail but also allows for better application of the acrylic material.

Finally, it is advisable to thoroughly disinfect the nail using a specific nail disinfectant to eliminate any bacteria or microorganisms present on the nail surface and prevent infections during the reconstruction.

By carefully following these preliminary steps, you can ensure a solid and clean base for acrylic reconstruction, guaranteeing optimal and long-lasting results.

2. Using Monomer and Acrylic Powder

Proper use of monomer and acrylic powder is essential for achieving a high-quality, long-lasting nail reconstruction. These two components form the foundation of the acrylic system and require correct handling to ensure optimal results.

Before starting, ensure you have high-quality monomer and acrylic powder in the desired shade. Monomer is a transparent or slightly colored liquid, while acrylic powder is available in a wide range of colors and textures to meet clients' aesthetic needs.

To begin the procedure, pour a small amount of monomer into a clean, dry monomer dish. Make sure to use a good quality acrylic brush with thin, flexible bristles, allowing better control over the application of the monomer and acrylic powder.

After preparing the monomer, dip the brush into the liquid and remove the excess by gently squeezing the bristles with your fingers. Then, pick up a small amount of acrylic powder with the brush and start working it onto the nail surface in an even and controlled manner.

During the application, ensure a uniform and consistent texture, avoiding excessive product buildup that could compromise the final appearance of the reconstruction. Work with precision and care to shape the nail into the desired form, using gentle and fluid movements to ensure a smooth and even surface.

Once the application of monomer and acrylic powder is complete, allow the material to dry thoroughly before proceeding with filing and final finishing. This ensures a solid and durable bond, guaranteeing impeccable and long-lasting results.

Always remember to follow the manufacturer's instructions closely and practice regularly to improve your skills and achieve consistently better results. With practice and the right technique, you will be able to create high-quality acrylic nail reconstructions and meet your clients' needs professionally and competently.

3. Acrylic Application Technique: Creating the Smile Line and C-Curve

Creating the smile line and C-curve is one of the essential skills in acrylic nail reconstruction. These techniques allow for a natural and harmonious look on artificial nails, giving them an aesthetically pleasing and comfortable shape for the client.

To start, it is important to have a clear understanding of the desired shape of the smile line and C-curve, which may vary based on the client's personal preferences and their natural nail type. Before applying the acrylic, carefully evaluate the morphology of the natural nails and discuss the client's aesthetic preferences.

Once the desired shape is determined, begin by applying a small amount of monomer to the nail bed and the free edge of the natural nail. This will help ensure better adhesion of the acrylic and prevent premature lifting of the product.

Next, use the acrylic brush to pick up a small amount of acrylic powder and start shaping the C-curve, working with gentle and precise movements. Apply the right amount of product to create a smooth and natural transition between the nail bed and the free edge of the nail.

To form the smile line, focus the application of acrylic on the free edge of the nail, gently shaping the desired curve with the acrylic brush. Ensure symmetrical work on both nails to achieve a uniform and balanced result.

During the process, constantly check the shape and appearance of the artificial nails, making any necessary corrections or adjustments to ensure optimal results. Work patiently and precisely, paying attention to details to create a flawless and well-defined smile line and C-curve.

Once the smile line and C-curve formation is complete, allow the acrylic to dry completely before proceeding with filing and final finishing. This ensures a solid and durable bond of the product, guaranteeing a natural and long-lasting look for the reconstructed nails.

4. Drying and Curing Acrylic

Drying and curing the acrylic are crucial steps in the process of artificial nail reconstruction. Proper drying and curing ensure a strong, long-lasting bond and a professional-quality finish.

Before proceeding with the drying and curing of the acrylic, make sure the previous work has been done carefully and precisely. Check that the shape and thickness of the acrylic are even on both nails and that there are no irregularities or excess product.

To dry and cure the acrylic, you need to use a UV or LED lamp specifically designed for this purpose. These lamps emit light at a specific wavelength that activates the photoinitiators in the acrylic, starting the curing process and hardening the product.

Before placing the nails under the lamp, ensure that all previous steps in the reconstruction, including forming the smile line and C-curve, are completed. Then, position the nails under the lamp and set the timer according to the manufacturer's instructions.

During the drying and curing process, it is important to carefully follow the manufacturer's guidelines and adhere to the recommended exposure times. Insufficient exposure can result in incomplete curing of the acrylic, while excessive exposure can cause overheating and damage the natural nails.

Once drying and curing are complete, check that the acrylic is fully hardened by gently touching it with the back of the brush or another non-sticky surface. If the acrylic feels solid and leaves no impression, the nails are ready for the next step in the reconstruction process.

Always work in a well-ventilated environment during the application and drying of the acrylic to avoid prolonged exposure to vapors and fumes. Additionally, regularly clean the surface of the UV or LED lamp to ensure proper functionality and optimal performance over time.

5. Finishing and Polishing Acrylic Nails

Finishing and polishing acrylic nails are crucial steps to achieve a flawless and professional final result. These procedures not only give the nails a smooth and uniform appearance but also help improve the durability and strength of the reconstruction.

Before starting the finishing and polishing process, ensure the acrylic is completely dry and hardened after curing. Any residual moisture or uncured product could compromise the final result and the longevity of the reconstruction.

To begin the finishing process, use a medium-grit file to adjust the shape and thickness of the acrylic. Work with gentle and precise movements, removing any irregularities and leveling the nail surface to achieve a uniform and harmonious shape. Ensure to maintain a natural and balanced shape, respecting the client's preferences and guaranteeing an aesthetically pleasing look.

Next, switch to a finer grit file to further smooth the acrylic surface and eliminate any marks left from the previous filing. This step is essential to achieve a smooth and even surface, ready for the polishing phase.

Once the finishing is complete, proceed with polishing the reconstructed nails. You can use a buffer or a polishing block specifically designed for this purpose. With gentle and consistent movements, pass the buffer over the acrylic surface to eliminate any imperfections and achieve a smooth, shiny appearance.

For an even more polished and refined result, you can use a three- or four-step buffer or polisher. These tools are designed to provide professional and long-lasting polishing, giving the nails a bright and glossy look that endures over time.

Always work carefully and precisely during the finishing and polishing stages, avoiding the removal of too much material which could damage the underlying acrylic. With practice and patience, you will be able to achieve stunning results and meet the aesthetic and functional needs of your clients.

6. Troubleshooting and Resolving Common Issues in Acrylic Nail Reconstruction

When it comes to acrylic nail reconstruction, being prepared to address any issues that may arise during the process is essential. Although constant practice and experience can minimize the occurrence of problems, it's useful to know the strategies for resolving common issues to ensure optimal results for your clients.

One of the most common problems in acrylic nail reconstruction is the formation of air bubbles within the acrylic itself. This can happen due to various factors, such as excessive use of monomer, an overly high ambient temperature, or applying the acrylic too quickly on the nail surface. To prevent air bubbles, ensure you work with the correct proportions of monomer and acrylic powder, maintain a controlled room temperature, and apply the acrylic with slow, even strokes.

Another common issue is difficulty in shaping the acrylic to achieve the desired form. This can occur if the acrylic is too dry or if the working time is too short. To solve this problem, work quickly but precisely, using the monomer efficiently to keep the acrylic soft and moldable for as long as possible. Additionally, you can use specific tools, such as acrylic brushes of various sizes, to shape the acrylic with greater precision and ease.

Other common problems include the separation of acrylic from the natural nail, premature breakage of the acrylic, and lack of adhesion of the acrylic to the natural nail. These issues can be caused by insufficient preparation of the natural nail, lack of adhesion between the acrylic and the natural nail, or improper application of the acrylic itself. To resolve these problems, make sure to carefully follow the steps for preparing the natural nail, use high-quality products, and apply the acrylic with care and precision.

In conclusion, addressing common issues in acrylic nail reconstruction requires patience, practice, and knowledge of the correct techniques. With constant practice and experience, you'll be able to successfully tackle any problems that may arise during the reconstruction process, ensuring exceptional results for your clients.

XII. Preparing the Natural Nail for Acrylic Reconstruction

1. Assessing the Condition of the Natural Nail

Before starting any acrylic nail reconstruction procedure, it is essential to conduct a thorough assessment of the client's natural nail condition. This preliminary phase is crucial to determine the nail's state and identify any issues or pathologies that could affect the reconstruction process.

The evaluation should include a series of methodical and accurate steps. First, observe the general appearance of the nail, checking for color, shape, and texture. Pay particular attention to any abnormalities such as structural deformities, discoloration, streaks, or thickening.

Next, examine the health of the nail by looking for signs of damage or infection, such as fungus, mycosis, or skin irritations. It's important to note any signs of breakage, peeling, or separation of the nail from the nail bed.

Additionally, assess the length and thickness of the natural nail, considering its strength and flexibility. This helps determine the amount of reconstruction product to apply and the best technique to use for optimal results.

Finally, take note of the client's daily habits and activities that could affect the durability and longevity of the reconstruction, such as manual work or sports. This information can guide decisions during the reconstruction procedure and in recommending home care products.

A comprehensive assessment of the natural nail condition provides a solid foundation for effective and long-lasting reconstruction, ensuring optimal aesthetic and functional results for the client.

2. Removal of Old Product and Nail Cleansing

The removal of old product and nail cleansing are fundamental stages in preparing for acrylic reconstruction. This process ensures that the nail is free from residues of previous products, oils, excess cuticles, and bacteria, providing a clean and safe base for the application of new acrylic.

To begin, it's important to gently remove the old product from the nails using a suitable file or an electric drill with an appropriate bit. During this phase, the technician must take care not to damage the natural nail underneath and avoid filing too deeply, which could weaken the nail itself.

After removing the old product, it's essential to thoroughly clean the nail and the surrounding area using a mild cleanser and a specific nail disinfectant. This step is crucial for removing any residue of product, oils, and bacteria that could compromise the adhesion and integrity of the reconstruction.

Next, it is advisable to gently push back the cuticles using a wooden or metal cuticle stick, exposing the entire nail bed and ensuring better adhesion of the new acrylic. Care should be taken during this operation to avoid injuring or damaging the cuticle and surrounding skin.

Finally, it is vital to thoroughly dry the nail using a sterile cotton pad or cloth to remove any liquid residues and ensure the nail is completely dry before proceeding with the application of the new acrylic.

In summary, the removal of old product and nail cleansing constitute a critical phase in preparing for acrylic reconstruction, ensuring a clean and safe surface to achieve optimal and long-lasting results.

3. Cutting and Filing of the Natural Nail

Cutting and filing the natural nail are crucial steps in preparing for acrylic reconstruction. These operations are essential to ensure that the nail has a uniform shape, is free of irregularities, and is suitable for the application of the new product.

Before proceeding with the cutting, it's important to assess the desired length and shape of the nail based on the client's preferences and lifestyle. It's advisable to use high-quality nail clippers or scissors and ensure to cut the nail straight or following the natural shape of the cuticle to avoid weakening the nail or causing any skin injuries.

After cutting, it's necessary to use a nail file to refine the shape of the nail and smooth out any rough edges. It's recommended to use a fine or extra-fine grit nail file to avoid damaging the nail and to achieve a smooth and uniform surface.

During filing, it's important to maintain a regular and gentle movement to avoid weakening or damaging the natural nail. Different filing techniques can be used, such as square, almond, pointed, or squoval filing, depending on the client's preferences and the desired outcome.

Additionally, it's important to pay attention to the cuticle during the filing process and ensure not to damage or irritate it. Using a soft nail file or buffer can gently remove any dry or thickened cuticles and soften the surrounding skin.

Finally, it's essential to thoroughly clean the nail and the surrounding area after cutting and filing, using a gentle cleanser and a specific nail disinfectant to remove any residue and bacteria.

In conclusion, cutting and filing the natural nail are essential steps in preparing for acrylic reconstruction, ensuring a solid and uniform base to achieve optimal and long-lasting results.

4. Preparation of the Nail Matrix

Preparing the nail matrix is a crucial step in acrylic nail reconstruction as it ensures a solid and durable base for the application of the new product. This phase requires attention to detail and precision to achieve optimal results and ensure the health and integrity of the natural nail.

The first step in preparing the nail matrix involves removing the cuticles and dead cells on the nail plate. This can be done using a gentle cuticle pusher or wooden stick to gently push the cuticles outward, followed by light filing with a fine-grit file to delicately remove dead cells and smooth the nail surface.

Next, it's important to assess the condition of the nail matrix to identify any irregularities or imperfections that could compromise the reconstruction. This may include grooves, ridges, or uneven surfaces that may require correction before applying acrylic.

For optimal preparation of the nail matrix, it's recommended to use a specific acrylic primer to enhance the adhesion of the product to the natural nail. The primer helps create a chemical bond between the acrylic and the nail surface, ensuring better adhesion and longevity of the reconstruction.

When applying the primer, it's crucial to ensure a thin and even layer on the nail surface, avoiding contact with the surrounding skin to prevent any irritation or unwanted skin reactions.

Finally, it's essential to allow the primer to dry completely before proceeding with the application of acrylic, thus ensuring a stable and adherent base for the reconstruction.

In conclusion, preparing the nail matrix is a critical step in acrylic nail reconstruction that requires attention to detail and the use of specific products to achieve optimal and long-lasting results.

5. Sanitization and Disinfection of the Natural Nail

Sanitization and disinfection of the natural nail are crucial aspects in nail reconstruction practice, as they contribute to ensuring a safe and hygienic environment for both the client and the nail technician. Before commencing any acrylic reconstruction procedure, it is essential to follow strict hygiene guidelines to minimize the risk of infections and contaminations.

The first step in sanitizing and disinfecting the natural nail involves cleansing the hands of both the client and the technician with antibacterial soap and water, followed by the application of an alcohol-based disinfectant to reduce bacteria and germs on the skin's surface.

Next, it is important to remove any nail polish or nail products using a specific solvent and sterile gauze to thoroughly clean the nail surface, ensuring better product adhesion during reconstruction.

Once the nail surface is cleaned, proceed with disinfection using a suitable nail disinfectant approved by health regulations. The disinfectant should be carefully applied to the nail surface using a sterile pad, ensuring complete coverage of the entire nail area and allowing the disinfectant to act for the recommended time by the manufacturer.

During the disinfection process, it is important to avoid contact of the disinfectant with the surrounding skin to prevent irritation or undesired skin reactions.

Finally, it is essential to maintain proper hygiene measures throughout the entire reconstruction procedure, such as using disposable gloves, sterilizing tools, and adhering to regular cleaning and disinfection practices to ensure a safe and hygienic working environment.

In conclusion, sanitization and disinfection of the natural nail are fundamental steps in acrylic nail reconstruction practice that must be performed with care and attention to ensure the safety and health of both the client and the nail technician.

XIII. Acrylic Application: Essential Steps

1. Preparation of Monomer and Acrylic Powder

The preparation of monomer and acrylic powder is a crucial step in acrylic nail reconstruction. Before starting any work, it is essential to ensure that all necessary tools and materials are available and to maintain a clean, well-ventilated environment for safe operation.

To prepare the monomer, use a clean and sterile container. Pour an adequate amount of monomer into the container, being careful not to overfill to avoid spills. It is advisable to use a dispenser to accurately measure the required amount of monomer, minimizing waste and ensuring proper mixing.

Once the monomer is in the container, it's time to add the acrylic powder. Use an acrylic brush to scoop a small amount of powder and add it to the monomer. Gently mix the monomer and powder with the brush until a smooth, lump-free consistency is achieved. Thorough mixing is essential to prevent the formation of air bubbles, which could compromise the quality of the final work.

During the preparation of monomer and acrylic powder, pay attention to the consistency of the mixture. The ideal consistency depends on the type of work being done and the personal preferences of the professional. Generally, a thinner consistency is suitable for more detailed work, while a thicker consistency is appropriate for stronger constructions.

After preparing the monomer and acrylic powder, it is advisable to cover the container with a lid to prevent monomer evaporation and contamination of the mixture. Also, make sure to clean the acrylic brush thoroughly after use to prevent hardened powder residue on the bristles.

In conclusion, proper preparation of monomer and acrylic powder is crucial for achieving optimal results in nail reconstruction. By carefully following the steps described and paying attention to the consistency of the mixture, you can ensure efficient and safe processing.

2. Acrylic Application Techniques: Wet Method and Dry Method

In acrylic nail reconstruction, there are two main application techniques: the wet method and the dry method. Both methods have their own characteristics and advantages, and the choice between them often depends on the personal preferences of the professional and the needs of the client.

The wet method, also known as "wet on wet," involves applying the monomer and acrylic powder onto damp nails. This technique allows for greater workability of the product, as the monomer helps to evenly spread the acrylic powder on the nail, facilitating shaping and creating a smooth surface. Additionally, the wet method promotes better adhesion between the product and the natural nail, ensuring greater durability and strength of the reconstruction. However, it is important to pay attention to the amount of monomer used, as excessive moisture can compromise the consistency and solidity of the product.

On the other hand, the dry method, or "dry on dry," involves applying the monomer on dry nails before adding the acrylic powder. This method is particularly suitable for professionals who prefer greater precision and control during application, as it allows for more precise shaping and results in a final outcome that is thinner and lighter. Moreover, the dry method is ideal for constructing nails with pronounced curves or specific shapes, as it enables the creation of defined and detailed lines. However, it is crucial to work quickly with the product once applied, as the monomer evaporates rapidly and may cause the formation of air bubbles or loss of adhesion.

In conclusion, both the wet method and the dry method are valid options for acrylic application in nail reconstruction. The choice between the two depends on the preferences and skills of the professional, as well as the specific characteristics of the job at hand. Experimenting with both techniques and finding the one that best suits your needs can help achieve optimal results and meet client expectations.

3. Shaping the Smile Line and C-Curve with Acrylic

Shaping the smile line and C-curve during acrylic nail reconstruction is a crucial process for achieving optimal aesthetic and structural results. These two characteristics impart a natural and harmonious appearance to the reconstructed nails, along with superior strength and durability over time.

To shape the smile line, which is the curved part of the free edge of the nail, it is important to employ precise and delicate techniques. Firstly, after applying the monomer and acrylic powder on the nail, the professional uses an acrylic brush to gently shape the upper part of the nail, curving it slightly upwards to create the desired smile line. Working with careful attention and precision is essential, maintaining symmetry between both nails and ensuring that the smile line has a uniform and harmonious shape.

The C-curve, on the other hand, refers to the curvature of the nail from the nail bed to the tip. To achieve a well-defined and uniform C-curve, the professional meticulously shapes the acrylic powder along the nail bed, ensuring to maintain a smooth and harmonious line from the nail bed to the tip of the nail. This requires a steady hand and a good understanding of the shape and structure of the natural nail.

Throughout this process, it is crucial to pay particular attention to symmetry and proportion, ensuring that the smile line and C-curve are balanced and seamlessly integrate with the structure of the natural nail. Additionally, considering the client's aesthetic preferences and adapting the shape and curvature of the nail according to their desires and hand characteristics is important.

In conclusion, shaping the smile line and C-curve during acrylic nail reconstruction demands technique, precision, and attention to detail. With diligent practice and a thorough understanding of shaping techniques, excellent results can be achieved that meet the needs and expectations of clients.

4. Drying and Polymerization of Acrylic

Drying and polymerization of acrylic are crucial stages during the nail reconstruction process. These operations ensure not only the proper solidification of the acrylic material but also the longevity and stability of the reconstruction over time.

After sculpting the acrylic on the natural nail surface, it is essential to ensure that the product dries and polymerizes correctly to avoid deformations, cracks, or premature detachment. There are various methodologies and technologies for drying and polymerizing acrylic, each with its own characteristics and advantages.

One of the most common techniques is air drying. After applying the acrylic on the nail, allowing the product to naturally air dry is possible. This method generally requires more time but is a safe and reliable choice to ensure complete polymerization of the acrylic.

Another option is the use of UV or LED lamps to accelerate the polymerization process. These lamps emit specific light that helps induce the chemical reaction that transforms the acrylic from liquid to solid. UV and LED lamps are widely used in beauty salons to reduce drying times and ensure rapid polymerization of acrylic.

It is important to carefully follow the manufacturer's instructions regarding exposure time and distance from the lamp during use. Additionally, it is advisable to periodically check the hardening of the acrylic during the polymerization process to ensure that all areas are properly solidified.

Another important consideration is the temperature and humidity of the environment where the drying and polymerization process takes place. Too low temperatures or excessive humidity can slow down the acrylic hardening process, while too high temperatures can cause deformations or cracks in the product.

In conclusion, drying and polymerization of acrylic are critical stages during nail reconstruction. By using the right techniques and equipment, it is possible to ensure complete and uniform polymerization of acrylic, thus ensuring long-lasting and high-quality results.

5. Finishing and Polishing Reconstructed Nails with Acrylic

Finishing and polishing reconstructed nails with acrylic are essential steps to achieve a flawless and professional final result. These phases not only enhance the aesthetic appearance of the nails but also contribute to ensuring the longevity and durability of the reconstruction over time.

The first step in nail finishing involves using files and buffers to shape and smooth the acrylic surface. Files are used to adjust the shape and length of the nails, eliminating any irregularities or protrusions. It is important to work with gentleness and precision to achieve a uniform and harmonious shape.

Once the filing phase is complete, the next step is polishing the acrylic surface. This process aims to impart shine and gloss to the nails, making them visually appealing and professional. There are several techniques and tools for polishing, including polishing buffers, three-phase polishers, and electric polishers.

Polishing buffers are used to remove any filing marks on the acrylic surface and prepare the nails for the next polishing phase. These buffers are typically available in different levels of abrasiveness, allowing for a smooth and uniform surface without damaging the underlying acrylic material.

After using polishing buffers, the actual polishing phase begins. This can be done using a three-phase polisher, which includes a series of polishing discs of varying grits to achieve a flawless final result. Alternatively, electric polishers that utilize high-speed rotations can be used to quickly and effectively polish the nails.

During the polishing process, it is important to pay attention to the pressure applied to the tools and the time spent on each phase. Excessive pressure or prolonged polishing can cause damage to the acrylic surface, compromising the final result.

In conclusion, finishing and polishing reconstructed nails with acrylic are fundamental steps to ensure a professional and long-lasting appearance. By using the right techniques and tools, it is possible to achieve an impeccable final result that meets the expectations of even the most demanding clients.

6. Troubleshooting and Resolving Common Issues during Acrylic Application

During the application of acrylic for nail reconstruction, encountering a series of problems and difficulties that can compromise the final result is common. However, with the right knowledge and correct techniques, it is possible to effectively address and resolve these issues, ensuring quality work that satisfies the client.

One of the most common issues during acrylic application is the formation of air bubbles within the product. This can happen for several reasons, including air incorporation during the mixing of monomer and acrylic powder or due to excessive movements during application. To prevent the formation of air bubbles, it is crucial to mix the monomer and acrylic powder gently and without creating abrupt movements. Additionally, working quickly and efficiently is important to avoid the product drying too rapidly, which can lead to bubble formation.

Another common issue during acrylic application is the formation of lumps or irregularities on the nail surface. This may occur if the product is applied in overly thick layers or if it is not worked on quickly and evenly. To avoid lumps, it is advisable to apply the acrylic in thin, even layers, working with precision and speed to distribute the product uniformly over the entire nail surface.

Another problem that can occur during acrylic application is product separation from the natural nail, also known as lifting. This can be caused by inadequate preparation of the natural nail, presence of oils or residues on the nail surface, or improper application of the product. To prevent lifting, it is important to carefully follow the steps for preparing the natural nail, ensuring thorough removal of any oils or products from the nail surface. Additionally, it is crucial to apply the product with precision and adhere to recommended drying times to ensure perfect adhesion between the acrylic and the natural nail.

Furthermore, issues related to acrylic discoloration, product consistency, or durability may arise. These problems can be addressed through the use of high-quality products, proper application techniques, and correct maintenance of the reconstructed nails.

In conclusion, addressing and resolving common issues during acrylic application requires knowledge, experience, and patience. With practice and attention to detail, it is possible to achieve excellent results and meet the needs of even the most demanding clients.

XIV. Advanced Techniques for Acrylic Reconstruction

1. Enhancing Nail Structure with Acrylic

Enhancing the nail structure with acrylic is a fundamental skill for every nail technician. This process not only corrects any structural defects in the natural nail but also creates a solid and resilient base for applying additional layers of product. Before beginning the reconstruction process, it is essential to carefully assess the condition of the natural nail and identify any areas that require particular attention.

The procedure starts with meticulous preparation of the natural nail, which includes removing any nail polish residue and pushing back the cuticles. Next, a light filing of the nail is performed to smooth out any irregularities and create a uniform surface. This step is crucial to ensure proper adhesion of the product to the natural nail and to achieve an aesthetically pleasing final result.

Once the nail is prepared, the acrylic structure is created. This is done by applying a thin layer of monomer over the entire nail and then picking up small amounts of acrylic powder with the brush and placing it on the wet monomer-covered nail. Using sculpting and shaping techniques, the technician molds the acrylic to create the desired shape and enhance the nail structure.

During this process, precision and attention to detail are important to achieve a uniform and well-balanced structure. It is also crucial to ensure that the acrylic is applied correctly and evenly to avoid the formation of air bubbles or cracks.

Once the reconstruction is complete, the nail can be refined to achieve a smooth and uniform surface. This may involve filing and polishing the acrylic to achieve a perfect and professional finish.

In conclusion, enhancing the nail structure with acrylic requires technical skills and a good understanding of the basic principles of nail reconstruction. With practice and patience, impressive and satisfying results can be achieved that meet the needs and preferences of clients.

2. Advanced Techniques of Acrylic Nail Art

Advanced techniques of acrylic nail art represent a fascinating and creative realm within nail reconstruction. This chapter aims to explore various methodologies and strategies for creating extraordinary and trendy decorations using acrylic as the primary medium.

One of the most popular techniques is three-dimensional acrylic sculpting, which allows for intricate and detailed designs directly on the nail. This process involves the use of small sculpting tools to shape acrylic into unique forms and textures, such as flowers, animals, or geometric elements. Color blending and adding details with acrylic paint or colored gels can further enrich the design, giving it depth and realism.

Another advanced technique is the incorporation of decorative materials into acrylic, such as glitter, sequins, or dried flowers. This allows for creating brilliant effects and interesting textures, adding a touch of luxury and originality to creations. It is important to learn how to properly manage these materials to ensure perfect adhesion and long-lasting durability.

The reverse method, or "reverse technique," is another option for creating high-quality acrylic nail art. This approach involves applying the acrylic layer directly onto a flat surface, such as a glass palette or adhesive film, and then removing and applying the design onto the nail. This allows for greater precision and control in creating complex and delicate details.

Lastly, techniques involving acrylic engraving and carving offer infinite creative possibilities for creating engraved or carved patterns directly onto the nail. This requires a steady hand and skill in handling engraving tools, but the results can be extraordinarily beautiful and unique.

In conclusion, advanced acrylic nail art techniques offer a world of possibilities to express creativity and talent. With some practice and dedication, it is possible to create spectacular and personalized decorations that will amaze and delight clients.

3. Use of Engravings and 3D Decorations

The use of engravings and 3D decorations represents a further evolution in acrylic nail art, allowing for intricate details and dimension to be added to creations. This technique involves the use of specialized tools to engrave acrylic and create incised or carved patterns directly on the nail.

To achieve optimal results, it is important to select the right tools, such as thin drill bits or scalpels, for precise control and delicate handling of the acrylic. Before starting, practicing on practice surfaces is advisable to become familiar with the tools and perfect the technique.

Engravings can be executed in a variety of styles and patterns, including geometric lines, intricate arabesques, or nature-inspired designs. This technique offers great creative freedom, allowing each design to be customized according to client preferences and current fashion trends.

3D decorations add an element of charm and dimension to nails, enabling the creation of impressive three-dimensional effects. This can be achieved using small decorative elements such as beads, rhinestones, glass beads, or gems, which are applied to fresh acrylic to create unique and eye-catching designs.

During the application of engravings and 3D decorations, it is crucial to pay attention to care and precision, ensuring that the added elements are securely anchored to the base acrylic and do not compromise the functionality or longevity of the nail reconstruction.

Finally, once the work is completed, it is important to carefully seal the entire design with a protective layer of clear top coat to ensure a durable and resilient finish.

In conclusion, the use of engravings and 3D decorations offers a wide range of creative possibilities to elevate acrylic creations, enabling the crafting of unique and breathtaking designs that are sure to capture attention.

4. Creating Special Effects with Acrylic

Creating special effects with acrylic is a sophisticated and engaging art form that allows for the addition of surprising and innovative elements to nail reconstructions. This technique involves using various advanced techniques to achieve unique and visually impactful results.

One of the most popular special effects is the marble effect, which recreates the velvety and layered appearance of natural marble on the nail. This effect can be achieved by mixing different shades of acrylic to create a marbled pattern, which is then applied to the nail and manipulated with specific tools to achieve the desired effect.

Another spectacular effect is the holographic effect, which adds a touch of brilliance and luminosity to nails. This effect can be achieved using holographic powders or pigments that create a rainbow reflection when exposed to light, giving the nails a sparkling and magical appearance.

Additionally, the translucent effect is highly appreciated for its delicacy and sophistication. This effect is achieved by applying a thin layer of transparent acrylic on the nail and incorporating decorative elements such as dried flowers or gold leaves to create an ethereal and refined look.

Another advanced technique is the incorporation of three-dimensional objects into acrylic, such as beads, glitter, or small jewels, to add texture and visual interest to the nails. This allows for the creation of unique and customized designs that stand out for their originality and creativity.

During the creation of special effects with acrylic, it is important to exercise precise control and accurate technique to ensure flawless results. It is advisable to practice on practice surfaces to perfect techniques and gain confidence in applying special effects.

Finally, once the work is completed, it is essential to seal the entire design with a protective layer of clear top coat to ensure a durable and resilient finish over time.

In conclusion, creating special effects with acrylic offers endless creative possibilities to elevate nail reconstructions, allowing for extraordinary and unique designs that are sure to capture attention.

5. Nail Reconstruction with Acrylic: Insights into the French Reverse Technique

The French Reverse technique is an innovative variant of the classic French manicure, offering a unique and creative approach to nail reconstruction with acrylic. This technique is distinguished by applying the white tip to the free edge of the nail, thus reversing the traditional look of the French manicure.

To achieve the French Reverse technique, it is crucial to follow a series of precise steps and use specific tools to achieve impeccable results. Firstly, preparing the natural nail involves removing the old product and thoroughly cleaning the nail. Next, the nail structure is created using monomer and acrylic powder, ensuring careful shaping to achieve the desired form.

Once the nail structure is complete, the French Reverse technique phase begins. During this step, the white tip is applied to the free edge of the nail, creating the characteristic white border of the French manicure in a reversed manner. This can be done using a pre-fabricated white acrylic tip or by manually creating the white edge with liquid white acrylic and white acrylic powder.

After applying the white tip, the nail bed is built using transparent or pink acrylic, ensuring a seamless integration of the white tip into the nail for a natural and harmonious appearance. This phase requires precision and attention to detail to ensure a smooth transition between the white tip and the nail bed.

Once the nail reconstruction with the French Reverse technique is complete, finishing and polishing the nail follows to achieve a smooth and glossy surface. Finally, a layer of transparent top coat is applied to protect and seal the design.

The French Reverse technique offers an elegant and modern interpretation of the French manicure, perfectly suited for a variety of styles and occasions. With practice and mastery of the technique, spectacular and refined nail reconstructions can be created that are sure to capture attention.

6. Setting and Crystal Applications with Acrylic

Setting and crystal applications with acrylic represent one of the most creative and appreciated techniques in the world of nail reconstruction. This technique allows enriching and personalizing nail reconstructions with the addition of crystals, stones, and decorations, creating unique and sparkling designs that capture attention.

To achieve setting and crystal applications with acrylic, it is essential to follow a series of precise steps and use the right tools. Firstly, preparing the natural nail involves removing the old product and thoroughly cleaning the nail. Next, the nail structure is created using monomer and acrylic powder, carefully shaping the nail to achieve the desired form.

Once the nail structure is completed, the phase of setting and crystal applications begins. During this phase, a variety of crystals, stones, and decorations can be used to personalize the nail design. These can be applied using gel or acrylic as an adhesive, depending on personal preferences and the preferred technique.

Settings can be achieved by placing crystals directly on the nail and then sealing them with a layer of clear gel or acrylic. This technique allows creating sophisticated and detailed designs, adding a touch of luxury and glamour to nail reconstructions.

On the other hand, crystal applications can be achieved by gluing the crystals onto the nail using gel or acrylic as an adhesive, thus creating customized and sparkling designs. Different shapes, sizes, and colors of crystals can be used to create unique and stunning effects.

Once the settings and crystal applications are completed, finishing and polishing the nail follows to achieve a smooth and glossy surface. Finally, a layer of transparent top coat is applied to protect and seal the design, ensuring long-lasting durability and an impeccable appearance.

Settings and crystal applications with acrylic offer endless creative possibilities, allowing the creation of unique and personalized nail designs. With practice and mastery of the technique, spectacular nail reconstructions can be created that are sure to attract attention and make a statement.

7. Carving and Sculpting Techniques on Acrylic

Carving and sculpting techniques on acrylic represent a refined art within the world of nail reconstruction, allowing for the creation of intricate details and stunning designs directly on the nail. This practice requires patience, precision, and a good dose of creativity to achieve extraordinary results.

To begin, it is crucial to have a good mastery of acrylic application techniques and nail structure creation, as a solid foundation is essential for successful carving and sculpting work. Once the basic structure is created, you can start exploring various carving and sculpting techniques.

One of the most common techniques is freehand carving, which allows for creating detailed designs using a thin brush and a metal or wooden tip. This technique enables the creation of intricate patterns such as flowers, leaves, animals, and other decorative elements directly on the nail, adding a touch of originality and personality to the design.

Another popular technique involves the use of molds or stencils for carving. These molds are available in a variety of shapes and designs and can be used to quickly and easily create complex patterns on the nail. Simply place the mold on the nail and apply acrylic inside the mold, then gently remove the mold to reveal the carved design.

It is important to apply even pressure during the acrylic application to ensure uniform depth and clear definition of the design. Additionally, using high-quality carving and sculpting tools is recommended to achieve precise and professional results.

Once carving and sculpting are completed, you can proceed with finishing and polishing the nail to achieve a smooth and even surface. Finally, apply a layer of transparent top coat to protect the design and ensure long-lasting durability.

With practice and mastery of carving and sculpting techniques on acrylic, you can create extraordinary nail designs that are sure to capture attention and make a statement.

8. Experimentation with Colors and Holographic Effects

Experimenting with colors and holographic effects opens doors to a world of creative possibilities in acrylic nail reconstruction. This technique allows you to play with a wide range of colors, shades, and reflections to create unique and captivating designs that stand out for their originality and beauty.

To begin, it's important to have a variety of high-quality acrylic pigments in a wide range of colors and finishes, including matte, glossy, metallic, and glittery. These pigments can be mixed and combined to create endless color combinations and effects.

One of the most popular techniques for experimenting with colors is the gradient technique, which allows you to delicately blend two or more colors to create a gradual and harmonious transition between them. This technique can be used to create multicolored backgrounds or to add details and shading to existing designs.

For achieving spectacular holographic effects, special holographic powders can be used that uniquely reflect light, creating a sparkling and brilliant effect on the nail. These powders can be applied directly onto wet acrylic or used to create three-dimensional details and decorations.

In addition to colors and holographic effects, you can experiment with a variety of decoration techniques, including the application of rhinestones, beads, sequins, and other decorative elements on the nail. These elements add a touch of luxury and glamour to the design and allow for the creation of customized and trendy looks.

To achieve the best results, it's important to apply the right amount of pressure when applying pigments and decorative elements and to use precision tools for achieving precise and clean details. Moreover, practicing on fake nails or artificial nails before experimenting directly on natural nails is advisable.

With practice and mastery of techniques for experimenting with colors and holographic effects, you can create extraordinary nail designs that are sure to capture attention and make a statement.

9. Using Pigments and Glitter to Create Unique Effects

Using pigments and glitter to create unique effects is one of the most surprising and versatile techniques in acrylic nail reconstruction. Pigments offer a wide range of vibrant and intense colors that can be blended together to create unique and personalized shades. On the other hand, glitter adds a touch of brilliance and glamour to designs, capturing light spectacularly.

To effectively use pigments, it's important to select high-quality pigments that provide even coverage and lasting results on the nail. These pigments can be applied directly onto wet acrylic for a rich and full effect, or they can be used to create details and gradients within designs.

To create a gradient effect with pigments, a delicate brushing technique can be used to gently blend two or more colors together, achieving a gradual and harmonious transition between them. This technique allows for creating multicolored backgrounds or adding details and shades to existing designs.

Glitter, on the other hand, can be applied directly onto wet acrylic or used to create three-dimensional details and decorations. You can choose glitter of different sizes and finishes, such as fine glitter, chunky glitter, or iridescent glitter, to achieve the desired effect.

For best results with pigments and glitter, it's advisable to use a precise application tool, such as a thin brush or a pointed applicator, to accurately control the amount and distribution of the product on the nail. Additionally, sealing the design with a layer of transparent sealant is important to protect and prolong the durability of the work.

Through practice and exploring different combinations of pigments and glitter, you can create unique and personalized effects that stand out for their beauty and originality, ensuring stunning and satisfying results for clients.

10. Techniques for Nail Reconstruction with Unique Shapes

Techniques for nail reconstruction with unique shapes represent a fundamental part of every nail technician's repertoire. Each client has nails with unique shapes and contours, often requiring the professional to adapt the reconstruction based on each nail's specific characteristics.

To tackle this challenge, it's essential to have a deep understanding of various reconstruction techniques and to be able to tailor them to the individual needs of each client. One of the most commonly used techniques is acrylic sculpting, which allows the technician to precisely shape the acrylic to create the desired nail shape. This technique is particularly useful for correcting damaged or deformed nails and for creating a solid base on which to apply gel or other reconstruction materials.

Another common technique is layering, which involves applying multiple layers of gel or acrylic to add volume and shape to the nail without weighing it down. This technique is especially suitable for creating long and slender nails or for adding reinforcement to weak or fragile nails.

For nails with unique shapes such as almond, stiletto, or squoval, it's important to pay special attention to the preparation of the natural nail and the modeling of the apex to ensure a uniform and balanced shape. This may require the use of specific tools, such as files and buffers of various shapes and grains, to accurately sculpt the desired shape.

Furthermore, it's crucial to consider the natural curvature of the nail and the architecture of the cuticle to achieve optimal aesthetic and functional results. This may involve using balancing and blending techniques to create smooth and natural transitions between the nail bed and the reconstructed nail apex.

With a deep understanding of reconstruction techniques and diligent practice, impressive results can be achieved even on the most challenging nails, ensuring satisfaction and confidence among clients.

XV. Finishing and Polishing Acrylic Reconstructed Nails

1. Importance of Finishing in Acrylic Application

Finishing represents a fundamental aspect in the entire process of acrylic application for nail reconstruction. This phase, often underestimated but crucially important, significantly contributes to the final quality of the work and the longevity of the application itself. Proper finishing not only enhances the aesthetic appeal of reconstructed nails but also plays an essential role in ensuring the durability and resilience of the acrylic over time.

During the finishing phase, any imperfections on the acrylic surface can be corrected, ensuring a smooth and uniform consistency. This step is crucial to ensure that the reconstructed nail has a natural and professional appearance, free from bumps, ridges, or irregularities that could compromise the final result.

Furthermore, finishing allows for precise shaping and defining of the nail, adapting it to the client's aesthetic preferences and ensuring perfect symmetry and harmony among the nails. This is particularly important when working with clients who require nails of different shapes and lengths, as it enables the technician to customize the outcome based on each client's specific needs.

Another reason why finishing is so important lies in preparing the surface for the subsequent polishing phase. A well-finished surface facilitates the polishing process, resulting in more uniform and brilliant outcomes. Additionally, proper finishing helps minimize the risk of damaging the natural nail underneath during the polishing process, ensuring the long-term health and integrity of the nail.

In summary, finishing is an indispensable step in acrylic nail reconstruction, contributing to the aesthetic quality, durability, and resilience of the application. A meticulous and attentive approach to this process will ensure satisfying results for the client and greater confidence in the technician's work.

2. Techniques for Filing for a Smooth Surface

In the process of finishing reconstructed nails with acrylic, filing techniques play an essential role in achieving a uniform and smooth surface. Proper filing not only enhances the final aesthetic of the application but also influences the durability and resilience of the acrylic over time. There are several filing techniques that can be used to achieve optimal results, each with its own characteristics and specific applications.

One of the most common filing techniques is the H-file. This technique involves using a medium-grit file to remove any excess acrylic along the edges of the nail, ensuring a uniform and symmetrical shape. Subsequently, a finer-grit file is used to smooth the surface of the acrylic, eliminating any roughness and irregularities. This process results in a smooth and polished surface, ready for the subsequent polishing phase.

Another widely used filing technique is the C-file. This method employs a curved file to follow the natural shape of the nail and remove excess acrylic along the free edge and sidewalls of the nail. The C-file technique is particularly effective in shaping the C-curve of the nail and ensuring a seamless transition between the acrylic and the natural nail. After performing the C-file, a fine-grit file is used to smooth the surface and achieve a uniform finish.

It is important to note that filing should be done carefully and precisely, avoiding overly aggressive or irregular filing, which could damage the natural nail underneath and compromise the final result. Before beginning filing, it is advisable to carefully assess the shape and thickness of the acrylic and plan the work according to the specific needs of the client.

In conclusion, filing techniques play a fundamental role in the finishing of nails reconstructed with acrylic, contributing to the creation of a uniform and smooth surface. With adequate practice and attention to detail, professionals can achieve high-quality results that meet client expectations and reflect the excellence of their work.

3. Using Buffers and Files for Nail Finishing

In the process of finishing acrylic-reconstructed nails, the use of buffers and files plays a crucial role in achieving a smooth and flawless surface. These tools help refine the shape and texture of the acrylic, preparing it for the polishing phase and ensuring a professional and long-lasting final result.

Buffers are essential tools in a nail technician's kit, as they gently yet effectively smooth the surface of the acrylic. Typically made from soft materials like sponge or abrasive fabric, buffers are used to eliminate any irregularities, round off edges, and achieve a uniform finish. When using a buffer, it's important to apply light pressure and move the buffer evenly across the entire nail surface, avoiding abrupt movements that could damage the acrylic or the natural nail underneath.

Files, on the other hand, are crucial for shaping the acrylic and defining the details of the reconstructed nail. Available in a variety of shapes and grits, files allow for precision and control, catering to the specific needs of each client. Coarser grit files are ideal for removing larger amounts of material and initial shaping of the acrylic, while finer grit files are used to refine details and achieve a flawless finish. When using files, it's important to follow the natural shape of the nail and work with gentle, controlled movements to prevent damage or trauma to the nail.

Another useful technique during finishing is the combined use of buffers and files. Starting with gentle filing to shape the desired form, one can then switch to a buffer to smooth the surface and achieve a uniform texture. This approach allows for progressive work, ensuring precise control and optimal results.

In conclusion, the use of buffers and files during the finishing of acrylic-reconstructed nails is essential for achieving a professional and high-quality finish. With practice and attention to detail, professionals can refine their skills in using these tools, ensuring satisfying and long-lasting results for their clients.

4. Steps for Professional Polishing

To achieve a professional polish on acrylic-reconstructed nails, it is essential to follow a series of precise and methodical steps. Impeccable polishing not only gives nails a shiny and refined appearance but also helps ensure the durability and strength of the acrylic over time. Below are the steps for effectively and precisely performing a professional polish:

Preparation: Before starting the polishing process, ensure that the acrylic is completely dry and polymerized. Check for any rough edges or irregularities on the nail surface, and if necessary, make corrections using a file or buffer.

Selection of Polishing Discs: Choose the polishing discs that are most suitable for the desired type of polishing and level of shine. Polishing discs are available in various grits and materials such as cotton, felt, or sponge, each offering a different level of polishing and finishing.

Application of Polish: Apply a small amount of polish on the surface of the reconstructed nail. Use circular and even movements to evenly distribute the polish across the entire nail surface.

Progressive Polishing: Perform the polishing in progressive steps, using discs with increasingly finer grits. Start with a coarser polishing disc to remove any imperfections and dullness, then move on to finer grit discs to achieve a smoother and shinier finish.

Checking and Refining: During the polishing process, regularly check the nail surface to ensure that the polish is even and free of scratches or marks. If necessary, repeat previous steps to improve the finish and achieve an optimal result.

Final Cleaning: Once the polishing is complete, remove any polish residue from the nail surface using a soft brush or a clean cloth. Ensure that the nail is completely clean and free of any traces of residual polish.

By carefully following these steps, it is possible to achieve a professional and high-quality polish on acrylic-reconstructed nails, ensuring satisfying and long-lasting results for clients.

5. Tips for Long-Term Shine Maintenance

To maintain long-term shine on acrylic-reconstructed nails, it is essential to adopt a series of precautions and practices that preserve the beauty and integrity of the reconstruction. Here are some practical tips to ensure lasting shine and impeccable nails over time:

Chemical Protection: Avoid direct contact with harsh chemicals such as detergents, solvents, or household cleaning products. Always wear protective gloves during activities involving such substances to prevent damage to the nail surface.

Adequate Hydration: Keep nails and the surrounding skin well-hydrated by regularly applying a moisturizing cream specifically designed for hands and nails. Consistent hydration helps prevent dryness and brittleness of the nails, contributing to preserving their natural shine.

Avoid Trauma: Be cautious to avoid trauma or impact on reconstructed nails, as they can cause chipping, cracks, or detachment of the acrylic product. Use appropriate tools for daily activities and refrain from using nails as tools for opening objects or lifting surfaces.

Regular Maintenance: Schedule regular maintenance sessions with a qualified professional to check the condition of the reconstructed nails and perform any necessary touch-ups or repairs. Regular maintenance helps maintain the shine and integrity of the reconstruction over time.

Avoid Exposure to Heat Sources: Protect reconstructed nails from excessive exposure to direct heat sources such as hairdryers, hair straighteners, or UV nail lamps. Excessive heat can compromise the stability and durability of the acrylic product, causing dullness or damage to the surface.

Use Specific Products: Opt for nail care products formulated specifically for acrylic, such as oils or strengthening treatments, which help maintain the shine and resilience of the product over time.

By carefully following these tips and practices, it is possible to ensure long-term shine on acrylic-reconstructed nails, preserving the beauty and elegance of a professional manicure.

XVI. Troubleshooting and Solving Common Problems in Acrylic Reconstruction

1. Perfect Planning: Avoiding Air Bubbles

When it comes to achieving flawless nail reconstruction, planning is crucial to prevent the dreaded occurrence of air bubbles.

These tiny adversaries can compromise the beauty and durability of the finished work, creating unwanted imperfections and affecting the material's adhesion.

The key to preventing air bubble formation lies in a series of precise steps and meticulous attention to detail right from the start of the reconstruction.

Before beginning the product application, it is essential to thoroughly prepare the natural nail by removing any residue of oil or moisture that could interfere with material adhesion.

Subsequently, the correct selection and use of products become crucial: from choosing the most suitable gel, acrylic, or acrylgel for the client's needs, to correctly mixing and applying the product on the nail surface.

The importance of proper application technique, avoiding abrupt movements that could trap air beneath the material, cannot be overstated.

Furthermore, proper curing of the product, adhering strictly to the recommended drying times and methods provided by the manufacturer, is essential to ensure a smooth surface free from air bubbles.

Finally, using specialized tools such as high-quality brushes and spatulas can further help reduce the risk of air bubble formation during application.

2. Brilliant Transparency: Resolving Opacity and Irregular Transparency

Uniform and luminous transparency is a fundamental requirement for high-quality nail reconstruction. However, issues like opacity or irregular transparency in the gel, acrylic, or acrylgel application process can sometimes occur.

The causes of these imperfections can be diverse and require careful analysis to identify the most appropriate solution. In many cases, opacity can stem from improper product mixing or the use of low-quality materials, while irregular transparency may result from application errors or impurities on the natural nail.

To address these issues and achieve brilliant transparency, it's crucial to follow a series of precise steps. Firstly, it's important to verify the quality of the materials used and ensure the use of high-quality products from reliable sources.

Next, meticulous attention must be given to properly mixing the gel, acrylic, or acrylgel, ensuring to strictly follow the manufacturer's instructions and avoiding the formation of lumps or air bubbles.

During the application of the product on the nail, it's essential to work with precision and gentleness, distributing the material evenly and avoiding excessive overlaps that could compromise transparency.

Moreover, using appropriate tools such as high-quality brushes and specially designed spatulas can help ensure even distribution of the material and reduce the risk of irregularities in transparency.

Finally, proper curing of the product is essential to ensure uniform and long-lasting transparency. By carefully following the drying times and methods recommended by the manufacturer, impeccable results and brilliant transparency can be achieved, showcasing the best of the reconstruction work.

3. Secure Adhesion: Eliminating Adhesion Issues

A crucial aspect of nail reconstruction using gel, acrylic, or acrylgel is the material's adhesion to the natural nail surface. Insufficient adhesion can lead to issues such as product lifting, cracking, or even complete detachment of the reconstructed nail.

To ensure secure and long-lasting adhesion, it's important to follow a series of procedures and precautions during the material application process.

Firstly, it's essential to meticulously prepare the natural nail by thoroughly removing any oil residue, cuticles, or other impurities that could compromise product adhesion. This can be achieved using specific nail cleaning solvents and applying adhesive primers that promote bonding of gel, acrylic, or acrylgel.

Next, it's crucial to apply the material evenly and without leaving gaps or air bubbles that could affect adhesion. Using appropriate tools such as high-quality brushes and spatulas can help ensure even distribution of the product and minimize the risk of adhesion problems.

During the polymerization or drying process of the material, it's vital to ensure that each layer is properly and fully cured. This may involve adhering to specific drying times or using UV or LED lamps to ensure optimal polymerization of the product.

Finally, it's important to educate the client on the importance of caring for and maintaining the reconstructed nails, providing advice on how to protect and preserve the work done in the studio. This approach can contribute to prolonging the reconstruction's durability and preventing adhesion issues in the long term.

4. Uncompromising Stability: Addressing Lifts and Detachments

When it comes to delivering high-quality nail reconstruction services, product stability is of paramount importance. Material lifts and detachments can not only compromise the aesthetic appeal of the work but also lead to discomfort and dissatisfaction for the client. Here are some approaches and strategies to tackle these challenges and ensure uncompromising stability in nail reconstruction.

First and foremost, it is essential to identify the underlying causes of lifts and detachments. These issues can result from various factors, including uneven material application, inadequate preparation of the natural nail, the use of low-quality products, or excessive exposure to moisture during the polymerization process. Once the specific causes are identified, targeted corrective measures can be implemented to prevent their recurrence in the future.

One of the primary strategies to address lifts and detachments involves employing enhanced natural nail preparation techniques and applying high-quality adhesive primers. These primers can enhance the material's adhesion to the natural nail, thereby reducing the risk of detachment. Additionally, using high-quality products and adhering to recommended drying times can contribute to greater durability and stability of the work.

In cases where lifts or detachments occur, it is crucial to promptly intervene to rectify the situation. This may involve removing damaged material, repairing the reconstructed nail, and applying new product layers. It is essential to communicate openly with the client and provide detailed explanations regarding the causes of the issue and the proposed solutions.

Lastly, to prevent future stability issues, it is advisable to educate the client on the importance of proper maintenance of reconstructed nails and provide advice on how to protect the work done in the studio. This may include using moisturizing cuticle oils, protecting nails during exposure to chemicals or harsh environments, and scheduling regular maintenance appointments for nail care.

By taking a proactive approach and adhering to best practices in preparation, application, and care of reconstructed nails, it is possible to ensure uncompromising stability and fully meet the needs and expectations of clients.

5. Resisting Cracks: Preventing Chipping and Breaks

When it comes to providing high-quality nail reconstruction services, preventing chipping, cracks, and breaks in the material is essential. These issues can compromise the aesthetic appearance of the work and cause discomfort to the client. Here are some tips and strategies to resist cracks and maintain reconstructed nails robust and durable over time.

First and foremost, it is crucial to ensure the use of high-quality products and meticulously follow the manufacturer's instructions during application. This includes proper mixing of gel, acrylic, or polygel, as well as adhering to recommended polymerization times. Accurate and uniform application of the material is essential to ensure a smooth surface resistant to cracks.

Additionally, paying particular attention to preparing the natural nail before applying the reconstructive material is important. This may involve removing excess cuticles, gently filing the nail surface to enhance adhesion, and applying a high-quality adhesive primer. Proper preparation of the natural nail can significantly reduce the risk of cracks and material breaks.

During the application of gel, acrylic, or polygel, it is important to avoid trapping air bubbles in the material. Air bubbles can weaken the structure of the reconstructed nail and increase the risk of cracks and breaks. To prevent air bubble formation, it is advisable to use a high-quality brush and apply the material in thin, even layers, avoiding sudden movements or excessive pressure.

Furthermore, educating the client about the importance of avoiding behaviors that could compromise the longevity of the work done in the studio is crucial. This includes refraining from using hard tools or objects that could damage reconstructed nails, as well as adopting proper nail care habits such as regular moisturization and cuticle oils.

Finally, scheduling regular appointments for maintenance and care of reconstructed nails is advisable. During these appointments, the condition of the work can be checked and any necessary corrections or repairs can be made. Maintaining consistent attention to the health and beauty of clients' nails will help ensure long-lasting and satisfying results over time.

By following these tips and strategies, it is possible to effectively prevent cracks, chipping, and breaks in reconstructed nails, providing clients with high-quality service and ensuring their complete satisfaction.

6. Impeccable C-Curve: Resolving Formation Issues

Creating an impeccable C-curve is essential to ensure the aesthetic appearance and structural stability of reconstructed nails. However, there are some issues that can arise during the formation of this curve, which could compromise the final result. Here are some tips and strategies to address common problems related to C-curve formation.

Firstly, it's important to carefully assess the client's natural nail shape and determine the most suitable C-curve type according to their style and preferences. A common mistake is adopting a C-curve that is either too pronounced or too flat, which may not harmonize with the natural nail shape. Ensuring clear communication with the client and understanding their expectations can help avoid issues with C-curve formation.

During the application of reconstructive material, particular attention must be paid to the curvature of the nail tip and the even distribution of gel, acrylic, or polygel across the entire surface. Using a high-quality brush and precise application technique can contribute to achieving a uniform and well-defined C-curve.

If problems arise during the formation of the C-curve, it's important to intervene promptly to correct the situation. This may involve partially removing the applied material and reapplying it using a more accurate technique. In some cases, specific tools such as tweezers or spatulas may be necessary to shape the C-curve more precisely and professionally.

Furthermore, educating the client about the importance of maintaining the C-curve during the nail growth phase is crucial. This may require regular application of nail care products and adopting appropriate lifestyle and care habits that promote the health and resilience of reconstructed nails.

Finally, scheduling regular appointments for maintenance and care of reconstructed nails allows monitoring the status of the C-curve and making any necessary corrections or adjustments. Maintaining consistent attention to the shape and structure of clients' nails will help ensure aesthetic and long-lasting results over time.

By following these tips and strategies, it's possible to effectively resolve issues related to C-curve formation and provide clients with professional, high-quality nail reconstruction services.

7. French Elegance: Perfecting the Technique

Perfecting the technique of French elegance requires meticulous attention to detail and mastery of application techniques using gel, acrylic, or polygel. The French manicure is a timeless classic that demands a steady hand and surgical precision to achieve impeccable results. Here are some practical tips to refine this technique and create an elegant and sophisticated look.

First and foremost, carefully selecting the right materials is crucial, including high-quality gels, acrylics, or polygels, as well as brushes and accessories designed specifically for French manicures. Using quality products ensures better adhesion, durability, and a flawless final appearance of reconstructed nails.

When applying the white color for the nail tips, it's important to maintain a crisp and uniform line. Use a thin and precise brush to draw the French manicure line with smooth and controlled movements. Also, ensure to apply a thin and even layer of white color to avoid unwanted clumps or streaks.

To achieve a perfect C-curve on the nail tips, it's helpful to employ a delicate yet firm "smile" technique. This method involves applying gel, acrylic, or polygel to the free edge of the nail with light and precise strokes, following the natural shape of the nail tip. Patience and precision are key to achieving a uniform and well-defined C-curve.

During the curing or drying phase of the white color for the French manicure, make sure to use the recommended polymerization time to ensure perfect adhesion and color durability. Paying attention to polymerization times is essential to avoid smudges or imperfections during the hardening process of gel, acrylic, or polygel.

Lastly, regular practice and experimentation with different French manicure techniques and styles are advisable to refine your skills and find the method that works best for you. Consistent practice and determination are crucial to achieving perfection in the French manicure technique and delivering outstanding and long-lasting results to your clients.

By following these tips and implementing the described techniques, you will be able to refine your French elegance technique and offer your clients a high-quality and professionally finished service.

8. Speed and Precision: Optimizing Drying

To achieve optimal results in nail reconstruction with gel, acrylic, or polygel, it is essential to optimize the drying process. The combination of speed and precision is crucial to ensure efficient and high-quality work that meets the demands of even the most discerning clients.

First and foremost, using high-quality products designed to ensure quick and even drying is important. Choosing gels, acrylics, or polygels with advanced formulas and optimized polymerization times will reduce overall drying times and enhance productivity during work sessions.

Another strategy to optimize drying is paying attention to the amount of product applied to each nail. Applying thin and even layers of gel, acrylic, or polygel ensures faster curing and greater resistance to smudges or imperfections during the hardening process.

During drying, it is beneficial to use a high-quality UV or LED lamp with optimal power and wavelength to ensure uniform and complete curing of the materials. Paying attention to following manufacturer's instructions and using the recommended polymerization time will yield the best results.

Furthermore, optimizing the drying process can involve using advanced techniques such as flash curing, which involves brief exposures to UV or LED light to partially cure the material and accelerate the overall drying time. This technique can be particularly useful when reconstructing thicker or more complex nails.

Lastly, regular practice and gaining familiarity with the specific characteristics of different products and drying techniques are important. With consistent practice and experience, you will develop an intuitive sense to determine the optimal timing to proceed to the next phase of the nail reconstruction process.

By implementing these tips and methods, you can optimize drying during nail reconstruction with gel, acrylic, or polygel, ensuring high-quality results and meeting your clients' expectations.

9. Safe Sensitivity: Managing Allergic Reactions

When working with gel, acrylic, or polygel for nail reconstruction, it's crucial to be mindful of potential allergic reactions from clients. While these materials are generally safe for use, some individuals may develop sensitivities or allergies to specific components. Therefore, adopting preventive measures to manage allergic reactions and ensure a safe working environment for everyone is essential.

Firstly, conducting a thorough allergy assessment with each client before starting treatment is important. Inquire if the client has experienced allergic reactions to nail products in the past and if they have known sensitivities to particular ingredients. Additionally, performing a preliminary skin patch test on a small area to check for any adverse reactions before proceeding with nail reconstruction is advisable.

During treatment, it's fundamental to use high-quality products free from harmful chemicals that can heighten the risk of allergic reactions. Choose reliable and certified suppliers offering products formulated with safe, dermatologically tested ingredients to minimize the risk of skin sensitization.

Furthermore, paying attention to signs and symptoms of allergic reactions during and after treatment is crucial. These may include itching, redness, swelling, or burning around the treated nails. If any signs of allergic reaction occur, discontinue treatment immediately and consult a physician for further evaluation and recommendations.

To further reduce the risk of allergic reactions, it's recommended to maintain strict hygiene practices during treatment. Keep all tools and utensils clean and disinfected, and adhere to personal hygiene guidelines such as thorough handwashing and wearing disposable gloves when appropriate.

Lastly, educating clients about potential allergic reactions and steps to take if they experience suspected symptoms is important. Provide detailed information about the products used, possible side effects, and advice on how to monitor and manage any allergic reactions at home.

With careful planning, the use of high-quality products, and open communication with clients, it's possible to effectively manage allergic reactions during nail reconstruction with gel, acrylic, or polygel, ensuring a safe and satisfying experience for everyone involved.

10. Cleanliness and Perfection: Removing Residues and Impurities

One of the crucial stages in nail reconstruction with gel, acrylic, or polygel is cleaning and perfecting the nail surface. Even the smallest residue of impurities or dust can compromise the durability and aesthetics of the finished work, so it's essential to pay special attention to this phase of the process.

To begin, ensure you remove any residue of old polish or nail art from the nail surface using a gentle, non-aggressive solvent. Use a cotton pad soaked in solvent to completely dissolve the old polish and gently remove it without damaging the natural nail surface.

Next, proceed with cleaning and disinfecting the nails using an antibacterial cleanser and a nail-specific disinfectant. Make sure to thoroughly clean both the nail surface and the surrounding contours to remove any residual bacteria, oils, or impurities that could affect the adhesion of the reconstruction materials.

Once the nails are thoroughly cleaned and disinfected, it's important to prepare the surface for the application of gel, acrylic, or polygel. Use a fine-grit file to lightly smooth the natural nail surface and create a uniform, smooth base to work on. Be careful not to file too aggressively to avoid damaging or weakening the natural nail.

After filing, it's crucial to carefully remove any dust or filing residue using a soft brush or a nail vacuum. Clean meticulously around the cuticles and under the free edge of the nail to ensure complete removal of any impurities.

Finally, inspect each nail carefully to identify any imperfections or areas that require further attention. Correct any irregularities using a fine-grit file or a drill and ensure the nail surface is smooth and uniform in preparation for the application of gel, acrylic, or polygel.

By following these steps and paying attention to detail during nail cleaning and perfection, you can ensure an impeccable and long-lasting final result for your clients.

XVII. Nail Reconstruction with Acrigel: Basic Concepts

1. Material Selection and Preparation

The proper selection and preparation of materials are crucial for achieving optimal results in nail reconstruction with polygel. Before beginning the process, it's essential to ensure you have all the necessary tools and products at hand. Firstly, having a complete polygel kit is important, including monophasic or triphasic gel, monomer, brushes of various sizes, tips or forms for extensions, files and buffers of different grits, primer, and base coat.

The quality of materials is another critical aspect to consider. Choosing high-quality products will ensure better adhesion, durability, and strength of the reconstructed nails. It's advisable to opt for reputable brands in the nail reconstruction industry that offer products tested and approved by industry professionals.

Before using the materials, proper preparation is key. Check that all bottles are tightly sealed to prevent products from drying out prematurely. Additionally, lightly shaking monophasic or triphasic gel and monomer bottles before use ensures a consistent texture.

Before proceeding with the application of polygel on the nails, it's essential to properly prepare the natural nails. This includes removing any polish residues and thoroughly cleaning and disinfecting the nails. Also, ensure to gently push back cuticles and lightly file the nail surface to promote product adhesion.

Once the preparation of natural nails and materials is complete, you are ready to begin the polygel reconstruction process. Follow the manufacturer's instructions carefully to ensure optimal and long-lasting results.

Accurate material selection and preparation are fundamental to the success of polygel nail reconstruction. Investing time and attention in this initial phase will guarantee professional and satisfying work.

2. Application of Primer and Base Coat

The application of primer and base coat is a critical step in polygel nail reconstruction, as it prepares the natural nail surface to ensure optimal adhesion of the reconstructive material and enhances the longevity of the finished work. Before applying any gel, it is crucial to follow a precise procedure to achieve professional and long-lasting results.

The primer is the first step in preparing the natural nail. It is a chemical product that dehydrates and primes the nail surface to promote gel adhesion. To apply the primer correctly, it is advisable to use a thin and precise brush to avoid excessive product waste. Apply a very small amount of primer onto the natural nail surface, avoiding contact with surrounding skin and cuticles. Allow the primer to dry completely before proceeding with the application of the base coat.

The base coat, or foundation layer, is the second crucial step in preparing the nail for polygel reconstruction. This layer acts as an adhesive base for the reconstructive gel, ensuring better adhesion and durability of the final work. To apply the base coat, it is recommended to use a flat and soft brush that allows for even distribution of the product over the entire nail surface. Apply the base coat in a thin and uniform layer, ensuring that the gel does not come into contact with surrounding skin and cuticles.

It is important to pay special attention during the application of the primer and base coat to avoid air bubbles, cracks, or premature detachment of the gel. Make sure to carefully follow the manufacturer's instructions and work in a well-ventilated environment to ensure proper application and drying of the products.

Proper application of the primer and base coat is crucial to ensure good adhesion and durability of polygel reconstruction. Investing time and attention in this initial phase will contribute to achieving professional and satisfying results.

3. Acrigel Construction Techniques

Acrigel construction techniques represent a crucial phase in nail reconstruction, as they allow for precise shaping and creation of the desired structure with strength and durability. Acrigel is a hybrid material combining the properties of both gel and acrylic, offering greater flexibility and longevity compared to individual systems. There are various techniques and approaches to working with acrigel, each with specific advantages and applications.

One of the most common techniques is the "boule method,"
which involves using small beads of acrigel to build the nail
structure. This technique provides greater control over product
placement and distribution on the nail, enabling customization
of shapes and lengths based on client preferences. When using
this technique, it is important to handle the product carefully
and work with gentle movements to avoid air bubbles and
surface irregularities.

Another popular technique is the "overlay," where a thin layer
of acrigel is applied over the natural nail to reinforce and
protect it. This method is particularly useful for strengthening
fragile or damaged nails and extending the longevity of the
reconstruction. During overlay application, it is essential to
distribute the product evenly across the entire nail surface,
avoiding excess that could compromise the final appearance.

Regardless of the technique employed, practicing and refining
skills are crucial for achieving professional and long-lasting
results. Acrigel offers a wide range of creative possibilities,
allowing for unique decorations, gradients, and designs that
meet the needs and preferences of discerning clients. With
patience, practice, and dedication, mastering acrigel
construction techniques enables the delivery of high-quality
nail reconstruction services.

4. Structure Consolidation and Leveling

Structure consolidation and leveling are two critical phases in
acrigel nail reconstruction, ensuring a solid and uniform base
for achieving an impeccable final result. These steps correct
any imperfections and irregularities, ensuring a natural and
professional appearance for the reconstructed nails.

During structure consolidation, it's crucial to ensure the acrigel layer is evenly distributed on the nail and properly adheres to the surface. This process involves using specific tools like brushes and spatulas to shape and mold the product into the desired form. Precision and careful attention are essential to avoid excessive buildup of material, which could compromise both the strength and aesthetics of the reconstruction.

Once structure consolidation is complete, the next step is surface leveling to achieve a smooth and uniform finish. This phase utilizes files and buffers to smooth out any rough spots and perfect the shape of the reconstructed nail. Working with gentle and controlled movements is important to prevent damaging the product and to create a natural and harmonious appearance.

Throughout both phases, paying attention to detail and working with patience and precision are key to achieving optimal results. Each step requires practice and dedication to master, but with experience, one can attain increasingly higher levels of perfection.

5. Finishing and Polishing of Reconstructed Nails

The finishing and polishing of reconstructed nails mark the final stages of the reconstruction procedure, yet they are equally crucial for achieving an impeccable and long-lasting end result. These steps refine the surface of the nails, eliminating any imperfections and imparting a glossy and smooth appearance.

To begin the finishing process, it's important to use high-quality files and buffers to shape and contour the nail according to the client's preferences. Working with precision and care ensures a uniform and harmonious shape, avoiding excessive removal of material that could compromise the structure of the reconstructed nail.

Once the finishing is complete, polishing follows to give the nails a shiny and lustrous appearance. This process can be carried out using polishers and buffers specifically designed for acrylic and acrigel nails. It's crucial to work with gentle and continuous motions to achieve an evenly polished surface, avoiding damage to the previously completed work.

Throughout both phases, attention to detail and working with patience and precision are essential to achieve optimal results. Each step contributes to ensuring a natural and professional look for the reconstructed nails, providing the client with a sense of confidence and satisfaction.

XVIII. Preparing the Natural Nail for Acrigel Reconstruction

1. Cleaning and Disinfection of the Natural Nail

Cleaning and disinfection of the natural nail are crucial steps in preparing for acrigel reconstruction. Before initiating any procedure, it is essential to ensure that the nail is completely free of polish residues, oils, and other impurities that could compromise the adhesion of the reconstruction material.

To ensure thorough cleaning, it is advisable to use a nail-specific cleanser or a mild cleansing solution that is acetone-free, as acetone can dry out and weaken the natural nail. Subsequently, thorough drying should be conducted using a sterile cloth or cotton pad.

Once cleaned, the nail should be disinfected to eliminate any bacteria or microorganisms that could lead to infections. A nail-specific disinfectant, preferably containing 70% isopropyl alcohol, ensures effective disinfection without compromising the quality of the reconstruction material.

It is important to pay particular attention to areas around the cuticles and beneath the free edge of the nail, where bacteria can accumulate more easily. Additionally, practicing proper hand hygiene before proceeding and wearing disposable gloves if necessary helps prevent contamination during the process.

Only after thoroughly completing the cleaning and disinfection of the natural nail are you ready to proceed with the next phase of acrigel reconstruction. Always remember that proper hygiene is fundamental to achieving optimal results and preventing potential complications.

2. Cuticle Removal and Surface Preparation

Cuticle removal and preparation of the nail surface are crucial steps to ensure effective and long-lasting acrigel reconstruction. Excessive cuticles can compromise the adhesion of the reconstruction material and create spaces where bacteria and fungi can proliferate, leading to infections and damage to the natural nail.

Before proceeding with cuticle removal, it is important to adequately soften them to make them easier to eliminate. This can be done by soaking the hands in a cuticle softening solution or applying a specific gel or cream for a few minutes.

Once softened, excess cuticles can be gently pushed back using a metal or wooden cuticle pusher. It is crucial to apply gentle and controlled pressure to avoid damaging the natural nail or causing bleeding.

Subsequently, with the help of cuticle nippers or a cutter, excess cuticles can be delicately trimmed and removed. It is important to take care not to cut too deeply to avoid injuries and bleeding.

Once the cuticle removal is complete, it is essential to prepare the nail surface to promote optimal adhesion of the reconstruction material. This can be achieved by lightly filing the surface of the natural nail with a soft file to remove the dull superficial layer and ensure better product adhesion.

Before proceeding with the reconstruction, ensure that the nail surface is completely clean and free from cuticle residues and impurities. Proper surface preparation will contribute to achieving long-lasting results and a smooth reconstruction process.

3. Evaluation and Correction of Natural Nail Shape

The evaluation and correction of the natural nail shape are crucial steps in preparing for acrigel reconstruction. Before applying any reconstruction material, it is essential to carefully assess the shape and structure of the natural nail to ensure a visually pleasing and durable final result.

To assess the shape of the natural nail, it is important to consider several factors including length, width, curvature, and overall appearance. A balanced and harmonious natural shape is fundamental for ensuring stable and long-lasting reconstruction.

During the evaluation of the nail shape, various irregularities or issues may be identified, such as nails that are too short, too long, too narrow, or too wide. It is important to recognize these imperfections and correct them adequately to establish an optimal base for reconstruction.

Various tools and techniques can be employed to correct the shape of the natural nail, including filing, cutting, and shaping. Filing is one of the most common and effective methods for shaping the nail, allowing precise and controlled adjustment of length, width, and curvature.

During filing, it is crucial to work carefully and gradually to avoid damaging the natural nail or creating irregularities. Using a high-quality file and following proper technique ensures consistent and professional results.

In addition to filing, other tools such as nail clippers or scissors may be used to address irregularities or excessive length. Precision and caution are key to avoid damaging the nail or causing discomfort to the client.

Once the evaluation and correction of the natural nail shape are completed, you can proceed confidently to the next phase of acrigel reconstruction, knowing you have a well-prepared and solid foundation to achieve optimal results.

4. Cutting and Filing of the Natural Nail

Cutting and filing the natural nail are two crucial steps in preparing for acrigel reconstruction. These stages are essential to ensure a solid and well-prepared foundation, promoting optimal adhesion of the reconstruction material and ensuring a visually pleasing and durable final result.

Before proceeding with cutting and filing, it is important to ensure you have the right tools at hand, such as nail scissors or clippers and files of various grits. Using high-quality tools is essential to achieve precise and uniform results while avoiding damage to the natural nail.

The first step is cutting the natural nail to the desired length. It is important to cut the nail evenly and follow the natural shape of the nail's apex. Using scissors or clippers designed for nails is recommended, avoiding cutting too close to the skin fold to prevent injury or discomfort to the client.

After cutting, proceed with filing the natural nail to adjust its length, width, and shape precisely and controlled. Filing helps to smooth the nail's surface and remove any irregularities or rough edges that could compromise the adhesion of the reconstruction material.

During filing, work gently and carefully to avoid damaging the natural nail or creating irregularities. It is advisable to use a high-quality file and follow an appropriate technique, working evenly and consistently across the entire nail surface.

Once cutting and filing are completed, you can proceed confidently to the next phase of preparing the natural nail for acrigel reconstruction, knowing you have a well-prepared base ready to achieve optimal results.

5. Nail Filing Techniques to Prepare the Natural Nail

Nail filing techniques for the natural nail are crucial to ensure a smooth and well-prepared surface before acrigel reconstruction. Proper filing not only enhances the aesthetic appearance of the nail but also promotes optimal adhesion of the reconstruction material and reduces the risk of premature lifting.

Before starting filing, it is important to carefully assess the shape and length of the natural nail, as well as the client's needs and preferences. Using a high-quality file with an appropriate grit size is recommended to avoid damaging the nail and achieve precise and uniform results.

A common filing technique involves using a horseshoe-shaped file, which makes it easy to shape and define the apex of the nail. Begin by filing the sides of the nail with gentle and controlled movements, maintaining a rounded or square shape depending on the client's preference.

Next, proceed to file the free edge of the nail to adjust its length and achieve a uniform and symmetrical shape. Work with care and precision to avoid damaging the nail or creating irregularities.

During filing, it is advisable to keep the file in continuous motion and avoid applying too much pressure on the nail to reduce the risk of damaging the nail's surface layer. It is also recommended to file in one direction, preferably from the outside towards the center, to prevent excessive damage to the nail.

Once filing is complete, carefully inspect the nail surface to ensure it is smooth and free of irregularities. Any rough spots or imperfections can be corrected with light additional filing until the desired result is achieved.

XIX. Acrigel Application: Essential Steps

1. Preparation of the Natural Nail

Preparing the natural nail is a crucial step in acrigel nail reconstruction.

Before beginning any procedure, it is essential to ensure that the natural nail is thoroughly clean and prepared to maximize adhesion and ensure lasting results.

Firstly, make sure to remove any residue of previously applied polish using a gentle solvent.

Next, carefully examine the nail to identify any signs of damage, such as cracks or lifting, which could compromise the final result.

In the case of damaged nails, it is advisable to consult with a professional to assess the situation and determine the most suitable treatment.

Once the nail has been inspected and cleaned, it's time to proceed with cuticle removal and surface shaping.

This step is crucial to ensure a smooth and uniform base for applying acrigel seamlessly and without issues.

Using a cuticle pusher and cuticle cutter, gently push back the cuticles and remove any excess skin to expose the lunula and the distal part of the nail.

2. Application of Primer and Base Coat

The application of primer and base coat is a critical step in the acrigel nail reconstruction procedure.

Before beginning the application of any products, it is crucial to properly prepare the natural nail to maximize adhesion and ensure optimal material retention.

The primer is used to prepare the nail and create a suitable surface for the acrylic gel to adhere to. It is a clear liquid applied with a thin brush onto the surface of the natural nail. The primer acts as an adhesive agent, helping the acrylic gel adhere firmly to the nail. It is important to apply the primer carefully and with precise movements to ensure even distribution and complete coverage of the nail.

After applying the primer, proceed to apply the base coat. The base coat is a thin, transparent gel applied to the nail to create optimal adhesion and a smooth surface to work on. This base layer also helps protect the natural nail and prevents the formation of spots or smudges during the application of the acrylic gel.

To apply the base coat, use an acrylic gel brush and apply a thin and uniform layer over the entire surface of the nail, ensuring complete coverage without creating lumps or air bubbles. Once applied, the base coat should be cured under a UV or LED lamp for the time specified by the manufacturer.

Be sure to pay special attention to this step, as proper preparation of the nail with primer and base coat is essential to ensure a durable and high-quality reconstruction.

3. Acrigel Construction Techniques

Acrigel construction techniques are a crucial aspect of nail reconstruction, as they determine the shape, structure, and longevity of the final work.

To begin, ensure you have all necessary materials at hand, including acrylic gel and UV or LED gel, primer, base coat, and working tools such as brushes and spatulas. Proper preparation of the workspace is essential to ensure precise and professional reconstruction.

Before applying acrigel, prepare the natural nail following the steps outlined in the preceding paragraphs. Ensure the nail is clean, disinfected, and completely dry before proceeding with gel application.

To construct the nail with acrigel, employ a layering technique involving the application of thin layers of gel to create a solid and resilient structure. Start with a thin layer of builder gel, which will serve as the foundation for nail reconstruction. Use an acrylic gel brush to evenly distribute the gel over the nail surface, ensuring complete coverage.

Once the first layer of gel is applied, cure it under a UV or LED lamp for the time specified by the manufacturer. This step is crucial to harden the gel and ensure a secure bond to the nail.

Next, proceed with applying additional layers of acrigel, gradually building the desired shape and thickness. Employ a layering technique to sculpt the nail and create a smooth and uniform surface.

Throughout the construction process, pay particular attention to the nail's shape and length, ensuring to correct any irregularities or imperfections as you progress.

Continue to work with patience and precision, adding layers of acrigel and shaping the nail until you achieve the desired result. Once the construction is complete, file and refine the nail to achieve a smooth and uniform surface, ready for final decoration.

As you learn and refine acrigel construction techniques, remember to practice consistently and be patient with yourself. With time and practice, you will be able to create high-quality nail reconstructions and meet your clients' needs in a professional and competent manner.

4. Structure Consolidation and Smoothing

After completing the nail reconstruction with acrigel, it is essential to consolidate the structure and smooth the surface to ensure a uniform and durable finish.

To consolidate the nail structure, use a medium-grit file to gently smooth the surface and remove any irregularities or protrusions. This step is crucial to stabilize the reconstruction and provide a solid base for the subsequent smoothing and finishing process.

Once the structure is consolidated, move on to the surface smoothing phase. Use a fine or extra-fine grit file to eliminate any bulges or imperfections on the nail surface. Work with gentle and controlled movements, ensuring not to remove too much material and compromise the nail shape.

During the smoothing process, pay special attention to areas around the cuticle and the lateral zones of the nail, where gel accumulations may form. Utilize an angled file or buffer to access these challenging areas and ensure the nail surface is uniform throughout.

Continuously inspect the nail surface as you work, using natural light or a LED lamp to identify any imperfections or irregular areas. Work carefully and precisely, gradually removing excess gel and smoothing the surface until achieving a smooth and uniform finish.

Once the smoothing process is complete, proceed to the finishing phase using a buffer or polishing file to achieve a polished and shiny surface. Ensure to work with delicate and even strokes to avoid nail damage and attain an impeccable finish.

Finally, thoroughly cleanse the nail with a cotton pad soaked in cleanser to remove any gel residues and prepare the surface for final decoration. With patience and attention to detail, you will achieve professional results and meet your clients' expectations with flawless nail reconstruction.

5. Finishing and Polishing Acrigel

After completing the construction and consolidation of the nail with acrigel, it is crucial to focus on proper finishing and polishing to achieve an impeccable and long-lasting result.

The finishing of acrigel is a critical step that helps define the shape and final appearance of the reconstructed nail. Use a fine or extra-fine grit file to gently smooth the contours of the nail, eliminating any irregularities and ensuring a smooth and uniform surface. Pay special attention to areas around the cuticle and the lateral zones of the nail, where gel accumulations may have formed during construction.

Once the finishing phase is complete, proceed to polish the acrigel to impart brilliance and shine to the nail surface. Use a buffer or polishing file to work on the surface with gentle and even strokes, removing any filing marks and achieving a smooth and shiny finish. Ensure to work carefully and precisely, avoiding exerting too much pressure on the nail surface to prevent damage.

During the polishing process, regularly inspect the nail surface to identify any imperfections or dull areas that may require further work. Use natural light or a LED lamp to highlight any defects and ensure you achieve a uniform and flawless finish.

Once polishing is complete, thoroughly cleanse the nail with a cotton pad soaked in cleanser to remove any gel residues and prepare the surface for final decoration. With patience and attention to detail, you will achieve professional results and meet your clients' expectations with a perfectly finished and polished nail reconstruction.

XX. Advanced Techniques for Acrigel Reconstruction

1. Enhancing Structural Strength

To achieve optimal structural strength in reconstructions with acrigel, it is essential to understand and properly apply a series of advanced techniques. The structural strength of reconstructed nails depends on various factors, including the correct preparation of the natural nail, precise application of materials, and careful construction of the structures.

Before starting the reconstruction, always ensure to perform a thorough evaluation of the natural nail to identify any structural issues or weaknesses. Preparation of the natural nail should be executed meticulously, including cuticle removal, surface leveling, and nail shaping according to the desired form.

During acrigel application, it is important to use the right amount of product and distribute it evenly over the natural nail. Pay particular attention to high-stress areas such as the free edge and sidewalls, ensuring the material is evenly distributed to achieve uniform structural strength across the entire surface of the reconstructed nail.

Furthermore, proper curing of the acrigel is crucial to ensure good adhesion and optimal strength. Follow the manufacturer's instructions closely for curing times and the use of UV or LED lamps to ensure complete polymerization of the material.

Finally, once the reconstruction is completed, it is advisable to apply a protective finishing layer to further enhance strength and prolong the lifespan of the reconstruction. Use a high-quality top coat and seal the edges well to prevent premature chipping and lifting.

Improving the structural strength of reconstructed nails with acrigel requires practice, experience, and attention to detail. With careful preparation and correct application of advanced techniques, robust and long-lasting results can be achieved.

2. Creating Complex Shapes and Designs

Creating complex shapes and designs is an advanced skill in acrigel nail reconstruction. This technique allows professionals to express their creativity and provide clients with personalized and unique results. To achieve complex shapes and designs, mastering the use of tools and understanding the basic principles of nail design is crucial.

First and foremost, it is important to have a solid understanding of the basic nail shapes and their proportional relationships. This provides a strong foundation on which to build more elaborate shapes. Common nail shapes include square, oval, almond, rounded square, stiletto, and coffin. Each of these shapes has specific characteristics and requires a different construction technique.

Once the basic shapes are understood, you can begin experimenting with more complex designs. These may include geometric shapes such as triangles, squares, and circles, or organic shapes inspired by nature such as flowers, leaves, and animals. Creating these shapes requires the use of specific modeling tools such as fine-point brushes, sculpting spatulas, and precision tips.

During the creation of complex shapes and designs, it is important to strike a balance between creativity and practicality. Highly intricate shapes may be challenging for clients to maintain in their daily lives, so finding a compromise between aesthetics and functionality is essential. Additionally, consider the compatibility of designs with the client's style and personality.

For optimal results, consistent practice and experimentation with different techniques and materials are recommended. Watching online tutorials, participating in workshops, and collaborating with other industry professionals can be helpful in expanding skills and discovering new ideas. With practice and perseverance, mastering the creation of complex shapes and designs is possible, allowing you to offer clients high-quality and personalized service.

3. Using Decorative Inclusions and Three-Dimensional Elements

The use of decorative inclusions and three-dimensional elements represents an exciting way to enhance acrigel nail designs, allowing professionals to create personalized and stunning artworks. Decorative inclusions can encompass a wide range of materials such as rhinestones, glitter, beads, dried flowers, gold leaf, and much more. These materials add depth, texture, and brilliance to the overall nail design, enabling the creation of truly unique and impressive creations.

Before applying decorative inclusions, it is essential to properly prepare the nail and apply an adequate base layer. This ensures that the inclusions adhere securely and durably to the nail, preventing premature detachment. Additionally, it is important to select high-quality inclusions suitable for nail reconstruction to ensure a flawless appearance and long-lasting results.

Once the base is prepared, you can begin placing decorative inclusions on the nail using tweezers or precision tools. Strategic placement of the inclusions is crucial to creating a balanced and harmonious design. This may require practice and patience, but the final result will certainly be worth the effort.

In addition to decorative inclusions, adding three-dimensional elements to nails can enhance visual interest and dimension. These elements may include charms, pearls, embedded rhinestones, pendants, and much more. Incorporating three-dimensional elements requires skill and attention to detail but can lead to extraordinary and unique results.

During the application of decorative inclusions and three-dimensional elements, it is important to ensure they are well-sealed with a protective layer of clear gel or acrigel. This helps protect the inclusions from wear and keeps them in place for a longer period.

In conclusion, the use of decorative inclusions and three-dimensional elements offers endless creative possibilities in acrigel nail reconstruction. With practice and experimentation, stunning designs can be created that will impress clients and showcase artistic skill.

4. Advanced Finishing and Polishing Techniques

Advanced finishing and polishing techniques are crucial for achieving a professional and flawless appearance in acrigel nail reconstructions. These techniques go beyond simple application of gel or acrigel and require a certain level of skill and attention to detail to ensure optimal results.

Before beginning the finishing and polishing phase, it is essential to ensure that the nail surface has been properly prepared and that each layer of gel or acrigel has been applied evenly and without imperfections. Any irregularities on the nail surface could compromise the final result, so it is important to take the necessary time to carefully prepare the nail.

Once the nail reconstruction is completed, you can start the finishing phase. This may involve using buffers and files to smooth out any roughness or protrusions and achieve a smooth and uniform surface. It is important to work delicately and precisely during this phase to avoid damaging the underlying natural nail.

After smoothing the nail surface, you move on to the polishing phase. This can be done using a series of steps with buffers and polishers to achieve a shiny and glossy finish. During polishing, it is important to work with light, circular motions to avoid overheating the nail and compromising the reconstruction.

In addition to manual finishing and polishing techniques, there are also electric tools and devices that can be used to expedite the process and achieve even more professional results. However, it is important to be trained in the use of such tools to avoid damage to the nail or surrounding skin.

Finally, once finishing and polishing are complete, it is crucial to apply a clear top coat to protect the reconstruction and prolong the durability of the result. This final layer also helps maintain the shine and brilliance of the nails for a longer period.

In summary, advanced finishing and polishing techniques are crucial for achieving professional and long-lasting results in acrigel nail reconstructions. With practice and attention to detail, it is possible to create impeccable and stunning nails that meet the needs and expectations of even the most discerning clients.

5. Insights on Correcting Errors and Common Issues

Errors and common issues during acrigel nail reconstruction can occur even for experienced professionals, but it's crucial to recognize and promptly address them to ensure optimal results. In this paragraph, we'll explore some of the most common errors and provide insights on how to effectively tackle them.

One of the most common errors is the formation of air bubbles in the acrigel during application. This can be caused by various factors, such as inadequate mixing of the acrigel or too quick application. To correct this issue, it's important to ensure the acrigel is mixed thoroughly and applied with slow, even strokes to avoid trapping air. Additionally, you can use a brush to gently remove any air bubbles on the nail surface before curing.

Another common issue is the formation of wrinkles or ripples in the acrigel during application. This can happen if the acrigel is applied too thickly or if the UV or LED light doesn't properly cure the material. To prevent this problem, it's important to apply a thin and even layer of acrigel and ensure it's fully cured with the UV or LED light. You can also use a spatula or brush to gently level the acrigel before curing to minimize wrinkles.

Other common problems include lifting or peeling of the acrigel from the natural nails and the appearance of cracks or breaks on the acrigel surface. These issues can stem from insufficient preparation of the natural nail, poor adhesion of the acrigel, or inadequate curing. To address these problems, it's important to perform thorough preparation of the natural nail, ensure proper application of primer and base coat to enhance adhesion, and carefully follow the manufacturer's instructions for curing and caring for the acrigel.

In summary, correcting errors and common issues during acrigel nail reconstruction requires patience, attention to detail, and familiarity with correct techniques. With practice and experience, it's possible to successfully address these issues and achieve stunning and long-lasting results.

XXI. Finishing and Polishing Acrigel Reconstructed Nails

1. Preparation of the Natural Nail

Preparing the natural nail is a crucial step to ensure effective and long-lasting nail reconstruction. Before beginning any acrigel application procedure, it's essential to dedicate time and attention to properly preparing the natural nail surface.

To start, ensure the nails are completely clean and free from any polish residue or oil. Use a gentle polish remover to eliminate any lingering polish from the nail surface. Next, proceed with cuticle removal using a specific remover or cuticle softening agent, followed by gently pushing back the cuticles using a cuticle pusher.

Once cuticle removal is complete, it's important to gently file the natural nail surface to smooth out any imperfections and create an even base. Use a fine-grit file to delicately shape the nail, avoiding harsh movements that could damage the nail bed.

Finally, it's crucial to thoroughly disinfect the natural nail and surrounding area to minimize the risk of infections. Use a nail-specific disinfectant or isopropyl alcohol to thoroughly cleanse the nail surface, ensuring it is completely dry before proceeding with the acrigel application.

Carefully following these preparation steps will provide a solid and clean foundation for effective and long-lasting nail reconstruction with acrigel. Paying attention to detail and dedicating the necessary time to prepare the natural nail is essential to achieving professional and satisfying results.

2. Application of Primer and Base Coat

The application of primer and base coat is a crucial step in the process of nail reconstruction using acrigel. These products play a fundamental role in ensuring optimal adhesion between the natural nail and the reconstructive material, as well as in protecting the nail and promoting the longevity of the final result.

Before applying any primer, it is essential to thoroughly prepare the natural nail as described in the previous paragraph. Once preparation is complete, proceed with the application of the primer, an adhesive product that enhances the adhesion of the reconstructive material to the nail. The primer is applied using a thin and precise brush, ensuring it is evenly distributed across the entire surface of the natural nail. It is recommended to allow the primer to dry for a few seconds before proceeding with the application of the base coat.

The base coat, or foundation layer, is the first layer of reconstructive material applied to the natural nail. Its purpose is to create a solid and uniform base on which subsequent layers of acrigel will be applied. Applying the base coat requires precision and attention to detail to ensure a smooth and even surface without air bubbles or irregularities.

Before applying the base coat, it is advisable to shake the product well to ensure it is homogeneous and free of lumps. Use a brush specifically designed for base coat application and apply the product in thin and even layers across the entire surface of the natural nail. Avoid overloading the brush to prevent excessive product buildup.

Once the application of the primer and base coat is complete, it is important to thoroughly cure the nail using a UV or LED lamp, following the specific manufacturer's instructions for the recommended curing time. Pay particular attention to ensuring complete polymerization of the material to achieve a strong and resilient base for the subsequent application of acrigel.

Carefully following these steps during the application of primer and base coat will ensure a stable and durable foundation for nail reconstruction with acrigel, minimizing the risk of premature lifting or detachment. Attention to detail and regular practice of these techniques will contribute to improving the precision and overall quality of the work performed.

3. Acrigel Construction Techniques

Acrigel construction techniques represent a delicate and sophisticated art that requires a combination of manual skills, material knowledge, and creativity. This process involves several fundamental steps, each contributing to the creation of a reconstructed nail that is durable, flexible, and natural-looking.

The first step in acrigel construction is preparing the acrigel itself. This hybrid material, composed of acrylic powder and gel, requires proper mixing to ensure a uniform consistency and effective polymerization. It is crucial to carefully follow the manufacturer's instructions for mixing acrigel, adjusting the proportions of powder and gel to achieve the desired viscosity.

Once the acrigel is prepared, the next step is its application onto the natural nail. This process requires dexterity and precision as the material needs to be evenly distributed over the entire nail surface, avoiding air bubbles or irregularities. Using an acrigel brush, the technician spreads the material from the cuticle towards the nail tip, working with fluid and gentle movements to ensure even coverage and precise application.

After applying the acrigel, the next phase involves shaping and sculpting the reconstructed nail. This process allows for defining the desired shape and length of the nail, working the material with specialized tools such as spatulas and files to achieve accurate and personalized results based on the client's preferences.

During the acrigel sculpting process, it is important to pay attention to the natural curvature and anatomy of the nail, ensuring a harmonious and comfortable shape for the client. This requires practice and mastery of sculpting techniques to create a final result that is aesthetically pleasing and functional.

Finally, once the acrigel sculpting is complete, the material is dried and polymerized using a UV or LED lamp. This step is crucial to ensure optimal adhesion of the material and extended durability of the nail reconstruction. Paying attention to the recommended drying time by the manufacturer and ensuring the acrigel is fully polymerized before proceeding to the finishing and decoration phase is essential.

As one learns and perfects the art of acrigel construction, it is important to dedicate time to practice and explore different techniques and styles. With patience and determination, it is possible to acquire the necessary skills to create high-quality reconstructed nails that meet the needs of even the most discerning clients.

4. Structure Consolidation and Leveling

Structure consolidation and leveling are two crucial phases in the construction of reconstructed nails with acrigel. These processes aim to ensure a solid and uniform foundation for the final decoration and finishing of the nail, contributing to its longevity and resilience over time.

Structure consolidation begins after the application of acrigel onto the natural nail and shaping it into the desired form. This step involves the use of specific tools such as spatulas and brushes to evenly distribute the material across the entire nail surface and along the nail bed. It is important to work with precision and care to eliminate any irregularities or protrusions, ensuring a smooth and uniform surface.

During structure consolidation, technicians may also focus on building reinforcement or raised areas, especially in regions prone to stress or breakage. This can be particularly beneficial for clients with weak or brittle nails, providing additional support and enhancing the overall strength of the reconstruction.

Once structure consolidation is completed, the next step involves leveling the acrigel to achieve a uniform and smooth surface. This process utilizes files and buffers to remove any imperfections, level the nail surface, and prepare it for the subsequent finishing and decoration phase. It is important to work delicately and precisely to avoid damaging the underlying structure and maintain the integrity of the reconstructed nail.

During leveling, technicians may also correct any misalignments or discrepancies in the nail shape, ensuring it is harmonious and well-proportioned. This requires skilled observation and a steady hand, but with practice and experience, impeccable results can be achieved to meet the expectations of even the most discerning clients.

In summary, structure consolidation and leveling are essential steps in the construction of reconstructed nails with acrigel. These processes contribute to establishing a solid and uniform base for final decoration and finishing, ensuring a visually pleasing and durable end result over time.

5. Finishing and Polishing Acrigel

Finishing and polishing acrigel are essential final stages in creating high-quality reconstructed nails, imparting a professional and impeccable appearance. These processes not only enhance the overall aesthetic of the nail but also contribute to its durability and resilience over time.

Finishing begins with the use of files and buffers to eliminate any roughness or irregularities on the surface of the acrigel. It is crucial to work with precision and care to achieve a smooth and uniform surface, removing any excess material residue and creating a perfect base for the subsequent polishing phase.

After refining the acrigel surface, polishing follows to impart a brilliant and glossy look to the reconstructed nail. This can be achieved using polishing buffers or shine enhancers, applied and massaged onto the acrigel surface until achieving a flawless, shiny result. It is important to work gently and consistently to achieve even polishing across the entire nail surface, avoiding scratches or accidental damage.

During polishing, technicians may also focus on specific areas of the nail, such as the free edge and cuticle area, to ensure a uniform and consistent final result. This may require skilled observation and a steady hand, but with practice and experience, impeccable results can be achieved to meet the expectations of even the most discerning clients.

Finally, once polishing is complete, applying oils or moisturizing treatments can nourish and protect the reconstructed nail, giving it a healthy and luminous appearance. This final step helps maintain the beauty and longevity of the reconstruction over time, ensuring satisfied and loyal clientele.

In conclusion, finishing and polishing acrigel are crucial final stages in creating high-quality reconstructed nails, imparting a professional and impeccable appearance. With the right technique and appropriate tools, brilliant and long-lasting results can be achieved that satisfy the needs of the most demanding clients.

XXII. Troubleshooting and Solving Common Problems in Acrigel Reconstruction

1. Adhesion Issues with Acrigel

When encountering adhesion issues with acrigel during the nail reconstruction process, it's essential to understand the underlying causes and effective strategies to resolve them.

Issues related to adhesion can stem from various factors, including inadequate preparation of the natural nail, residues of oils or fats on the nail surface, or improper application of the product.

To ensure proper adhesion of acrigel, it's crucial to follow a meticulous preparation procedure, which includes cleaning and degreasing the nail, as well as properly applying primer to enhance material adherence.

Furthermore, it's important to ensure that the acrigel layer is applied evenly and without air bubbles, using appropriate application techniques.

In cases where adhesion issues arise, they can be corrected by applying additional layers of primer or by removing and refinishing the affected area.

By adopting careful methodology and adhering to recommended procedures, it is possible to successfully address acrigel adhesion issues, ensuring high-quality and long-lasting results.

2. Opacity and Irregular Transparency of Acrigel

When facing issues of opacity or irregular transparency with acrigel during the nail reconstruction process, it's important to identify potential causes and apply necessary corrections to achieve optimal results.

The presence of opacity or irregular transparency can stem from various factors, including the quality of materials used, improper application of the product, or inadequate preparation of the natural nail.

To ensure proper opacity and transparency of acrigel, it's essential to use high-quality products and carefully follow their application instructions. Additionally, it's important to ensure that the natural nail has been properly prepared by removing any residues of oils or previously applied products.

During the application of acrigel, it's crucial to work in thin and uniform layers, avoiding excessive product buildup that could compromise the transparency of the final result.

If issues of opacity or irregular transparency arise, they can be corrected by applying additional thin layers of acrigel or by removing and refinishing the affected area.

By adopting a precise methodology and using quality products, it's possible to achieve uniform application and a transparent, glossy finish with acrigel, ensuring satisfying and long-lasting results.

3. Breakage and Lifting of Acrigel

Breakage and lifting of acrigel can pose a common challenge during the nail reconstruction process, but with the right techniques and precautions, they can be effectively prevented and managed.

Breakage of acrigel can occur due to various factors, including improper application of the product, excessive exposure to moisture during curing, or inadequate preparation of the natural nail. It's crucial to ensure that acrigel is applied in even layers and properly cured to ensure its strength and durability. Additionally, thorough preparation of the natural nail by removing any oily residues and using suitable products to enhance adhesion is essential.

Lifting of acrigel can happen when the product separates from the natural nail due to insufficient adhesion or trapped air under the gel. To prevent lifting, it's important to apply the gel evenly, avoiding air bubbles and ensuring proper adhesion to the nail surface. It's also advisable to carefully seal the edges of the gel to prevent excessive water ingress that could cause lifting over time.

In case of breakage or lifting of acrigel, prompt intervention is crucial to repair the nail and prevent further damage. This can be achieved by gently removing the damaged gel, addressing any imperfections in the natural nail, and reapplying the gel correctly.

In summary, preventing and managing breakage and lifting of acrigel requires a combination of meticulous preparation, proper application, and timely intervention. With practice and mastery of appropriate techniques, it's possible to ensure stable and durable application of acrigel, achieving professional and satisfying results.

4. Cracks and Fractures of Acrigel

Cracks and fractures of acrigel can be common issues during nail reconstruction and require special attention to ensure optimal and lasting results.

Cracks can occur due to various factors, such as excessively thick application or excessive bending of the nail. It's important to apply acrigel in thin and even layers to avoid excessive stress on the nail surface. Additionally, ensuring that each layer is properly cured with a UV or LED lamp is essential to achieve a strong and resilient bond.

Fractures can happen when acrigel experiences trauma or external pressure, causing the material to break. To prevent fractures, it's advisable to avoid activities that could expose the nails to excessive stress, such as using nails as tools or prolonged contact with harsh chemicals.

In case cracks or fractures occur, prompt intervention is crucial to prevent further damage and restore the nail's integrity. This can be achieved by gently removing the damaged gel, filling any gaps with new acrigel material, and sealing the surface carefully to prevent water infiltration and further damage.

It's also important to educate the client on the importance of proper maintenance of reconstructed nails and provide advice on how to avoid situations that could lead to cracks or fractures.

In conclusion, preventing and managing cracks and fractures of acrigel requires a combination of correct application, adequate maintenance, and timely intervention in case of damage. With practice and experience, it's possible to achieve professional and long-lasting results that meet the clients' needs.

5. Air Bubbles Formation in Acrigel

The formation of air bubbles in acrigel is a common issue that can compromise the appearance and durability of reconstructed nails. These bubbles may appear as small surface imperfections or more noticeable deformations within the acrigel material, creating an unattractive effect and compromising the structural strength of the nail.

Air bubbles can result from various causes, including poor preparation of the natural nail, too rapid application of the product, or the use of inappropriate tools during the reconstruction process. Therefore, dedicating time to prepare the natural nail by thoroughly removing any oils and residues through gentle filing and meticulous cleaning is essential.

During the application of acrigel, it's crucial to work with precision and patience, avoiding abrupt movements that could trap air within the gel. Using thin and uniform layers of acrigel and ensuring the product is evenly spread over the entire nail surface helps to prevent buildup and creates a solid foundation.

Moreover, it's advisable to use a high-quality brush and employ gentle, controlled strokes to evenly distribute the gel on the nail. Avoid vigorously shaking or over-mixing the product during application, as this could introduce air into the gel and promote bubble formation.

If air bubbles do appear during application, they can be corrected using a specially designed brush to push the air out of the gel before it fully cures. Subsequently, gently leveling the surface with a light filing ensures a smooth, defect-free finish.

In conclusion, preventing the formation of air bubbles requires attention to detail and accurate technique during acrigel application. With practice and a proper understanding of techniques, achieving a flawless, professional result that meets the needs of even the most discerning clients is possible.

XXIII. Tips for Maintaining Reconstructed Nails

1. Daily Hygiene and Cleaning

Proper hygiene and daily cleaning of reconstructed nails are essential for maintaining their long-term health and beauty.

Before starting any cleaning procedure, ensure you have all the necessary tools ready, such as nail brushes, gentle cleansers, and optionally disinfectant solutions.

To begin, carefully remove any nail polish residue or dirt using a mild solvent, avoiding scratching or damaging the nail surface.

Next, soak your hands in warm water with soap or gentle detergent for a few minutes to soften the skin and cuticles. Use a nail brush to gently clean around the nails, removing any accumulated dirt or product residues.

After thoroughly drying your hands, apply a specific cuticle and nail moisturizer to keep the skin soft and hydrated.

It's important to perform this cleaning and hygiene routine regularly, preferably at least once a day, to prevent dirt and bacteria buildup that could compromise nail health.

2. Protection from External Aggressions

Protecting reconstructed nails from external aggressors is essential to maintain optimal conditions and prevent undesired damage.

To safeguard nails from external aggressors, it's advisable to use gloves when engaging in household chores or manual work that may expose nails to chemicals or physical impacts. Gloves should be made from durable and waterproof materials to ensure effective protection.

Additionally, avoid using reconstructed nails as tools to open or scratch hard surfaces like boxes or packages, as this could cause damage to the nail surface or even break the reconstructed material.

It's also prudent to be cautious during activities involving water, such as dishwashing or bathing, as prolonged exposure to water and moisture can weaken the bond between the acrigel and the natural nail, increasing the risk of lifting or breakage.

Furthermore, refrain from exposing reconstructed nails to excessive heat sources such as hair dryers or UV lamps, as this could compromise the material's stability and cause irreversible damage.

Finally, consider using specific products for the care and protection of reconstructed nails, such as strengthening oils or polishes, to provide an additional layer of protection and nourishment to the nail surface.

By following these precautions and practicing proper maintenance, you can ensure that reconstructed nails remain strong, healthy, and beautiful over time.

3. Nutrition and Hydration of Nails

Proper nutrition and hydration of nails are essential to keep them strong, flexible, and healthy. Like any other part of the body, nails require specific nutrients to grow and remain robust over time.

Firstly, it's important to maintain a balanced diet rich in nutrients to ensure an adequate intake of essential vitamins and minerals for nail health. Some particularly important nutrients include biotin, vitamin E, calcium, zinc, and proteins. These nutrients promote nail growth, improve their strength, and reduce brittleness.

For instance, biotin is known to promote nail and hair growth and can be found in foods such as eggs, nuts, avocados, and bananas. Vitamin E is a powerful antioxidant that helps protect nails from environmental damage and can be found in foods like almonds, spinach, and sunflower seeds.

Moreover, maintaining adequate hydration is crucial for nail health. Water helps to keep nails and the surrounding skin hydrated, preventing dryness and brittleness. Drinking at least eight glasses of water a day can help keep nails hydrated and flexible.

In addition to diet and hydration, regularly applying oils and moisturizing creams specifically formulated for nails can help maintain their elasticity and strength. Natural oils such as coconut oil, sweet almond oil, and jojoba oil can be massaged onto nails and cuticles to nourish and moisturize the surrounding area.

In conclusion, proper nutrition, hydration, and care of nails are essential to keep them healthy and beautiful over time. Incorporating a balanced diet with nutrient-rich foods, drinking plenty of water, and using moisturizing oils and creams can help maintain strong, flexible, and resilient nails.

4. Monitoring the Health Status of Nails

Regularly monitoring the health status of nails is an important habit to promptly identify any issues and take necessary measures to maintain optimal conditions. Carefully examining nails can provide valuable insights into the overall health of the body and reveal signs of nutritional deficiencies, underlying health issues, or environmental damage.

During monitoring, it is essential to observe various aspects of the nails, including color, shape, thickness, texture, and integrity. A sudden change in nail color, for example, could indicate health issues such as vitamin deficiencies, fungal infections, or circulation problems. Yellowish nails might signify a fungal infection, while a bluish hue could indicate circulation issues.

The shape and thickness of nails can also offer clues about health status. Thin and brittle nails may indicate nutritional deficiencies or underlying medical conditions, whereas thick and opaque nails could be signs of fungal infections or nail psoriasis.

Texture is another important aspect to consider during monitoring. Irregular or deeply grooved nails could indicate health problems such as eczema, psoriasis, or thyroid issues. Additionally, the presence of white spots or patches on nails might signal physical damage or nutritional deficiencies.

Lastly, it is crucial to pay attention to any damage or structural abnormalities on the nails. Frequent nail breakage or lifting of reconstructed material may indicate the use of inappropriate products or improper application techniques. Moreover, the formation of cracks, fractures, or distortions in acrylic gel may require thorough assessment and correction to prevent further damage or infections.

In conclusion, regular monitoring of the health status of nails is essential to promptly detect any issues and take necessary actions to maintain their health. Carefully observing the color, shape, thickness, texture, and integrity of nails can provide valuable insights into the overall health of the body and prevent potential complications.

5. Tips to Prolong the Longevity of Nail Reconstruction

To extend the longevity of nail reconstruction with acrylic gel, it is crucial to adopt a series of precautions and follow daily maintenance practices. Properly adhering to these suggestions can significantly preserve the appearance and strength of the reconstructed nails, ensuring optimal durability of the work done.

First and foremost, it's important to avoid exposure to harsh chemicals that could damage or compromise the integrity of the acrylic gel. These substances include household cleaners, nail polish removers, industrial cleaning products, and corrosive substances. Protecting hands with gloves during exposure to such agents can help prevent damage to the nail reconstruction.

Additionally, it is advisable to refrain from using reconstructed nails excessively as tools for opening or scratching objects. Artificial nails, when subjected to excessive mechanical stress, can more easily become damaged or detached. Use appropriate tools for heavy tasks and handle your nails with care to avoid premature damage.

Proper nail hydration is another crucial aspect to maintain the longevity of the reconstruction. Regularly applying oils or specific nail moisturizers can help maintain the flexibility and strength of the acrylic gel, reducing the risk of breakage or lifting. Furthermore, it is advisable to avoid prolonged exposure to water or detergents, as excessive moisture can weaken the adhesion of acrylic gel to natural nails.

Finally, scheduling regular maintenance appointments with a qualified nail reconstruction professional is recommended. During these visits, the technician can conduct regular checks, perform necessary touch-ups, and assess the overall condition of the nails. Additionally, maintenance sessions can include reinforcement treatments or reconstruction renewals to ensure longevity over time.

Carefully following these tips can significantly contribute to prolonging the longevity of nail reconstruction with acrylic gel, maintaining impeccable appearance and optimal strength over time.

XXIV. Marketing and Promotion Tips for Nail Technician Services

1. Identifying the Target Customer Base

Identifying the target customer base is a fundamental step for success in the nail technician industry. This process involves analyzing and understanding the demographic, behavioral, and psychographic characteristics of the audience you want to target with your services.

Initially, it's essential to define the type of customers you aim to attract, considering factors such as age, gender, occupation, interests, and lifestyle. For example, if your target is a younger, trendier audience, adopting an innovative and creative approach in promoting your services may be necessary. On the other hand, if your focus is on more mature and professional clients, communicating an image of reliability and competence could be important.

In addition to demographic characteristics, understanding the needs, desires, and concerns of your target customer base is equally crucial. This can be achieved through market research, surveys, interviews, and direct observations. For instance, discovering that many potential clients are interested in treatments to strengthen weak or damaged nails allows you to tailor your offerings to address this specific issue.

Furthermore, considering the geographical and cultural context in which you operate is helpful, as customer preferences and needs can vary based on region or country. Ultimately, accurate identification of the target customer base provides a solid foundation for developing targeted and effective marketing strategies. These strategies enable you to reach and best satisfy customer needs, thereby enhancing the success and growth of your business.

2. Branding Strategies and Market Positioning

Developing branding strategies and positioning in the market are crucial for standing out from the competition and creating a distinctive, recognizable image for your nail technician studio.

One of the initial considerations is creating a captivating and memorable business name that reflects the brand's identity and values. This name should be easy to pronounce, easily memorable, and not easily confused with other names already in the market. Additionally, it's important to check the availability of the name for the website domain and on major social media platforms to ensure a consistent and uniform online presence.

Next, it's essential to develop a distinctive and professional logo that visually represents the brand. The logo should align with the desired style and image and may include elements such as symbols, colors, and fonts that convey the essence of the brand. Once created, the logo should be used across all marketing materials, including business cards, brochures, websites, and social media profiles, to ensure consistency and brand recognition across all communication channels.

Simultaneously, defining a unique and compelling value proposition is essential—what makes your nail technician studio different and better than the competition. This could include aspects such as service quality, staff expertise, use of high-quality products, or exceptional customer care. Clearly communicating this value proposition through all marketing materials will help capture the attention of potential customers and differentiate your studio in the market.

Finally, developing an effective communication and promotion strategy is important for increasing visibility and attractiveness of your brand. This could involve activities such as social media advertising, collaborations with industry influencers, participation in trade fairs and events, promotional offers, and customer loyalty programs. Investing in these marketing activities can help increase brand awareness, generate interest, and attract new customers to your nail technician studio.

3. Utilizing Social Media for Promotion

The use of social media has become a fundamental tool for effectively promoting nail technician services. However, to achieve positive results, it's crucial to adopt a well-defined and personalized strategy that considers the specific needs and target audience of your studio.

Firstly, it's important to identify the most appropriate social media platforms to reach your target clientele. Popular platforms such as Instagram, Facebook, and Pinterest are often common choices for nail technicians because they allow sharing captivating photos and videos of their work and direct interaction with potential and existing clients.

Once the most suitable social media platforms are chosen, it's essential to create engaging and high-quality content that captures the audience's attention and reflects the image and style of your brand. This content may include nail art photos, video tutorials on nail reconstruction techniques, nail care and maintenance tips, as well as behind-the-scenes glimpses of your studio and daily work.

Moreover, maintaining an active and engaging presence on social media is important. Respond promptly to comments and messages from clients, participate in community conversations, and regularly share content. This helps build a closer relationship with the audience and develops a sense of trust and affinity with the brand.

In addition to organic content creation, leveraging advertising features offered by social media platforms can effectively promote your nail technician services. Targeted advertising campaigns enable reaching specific audience segments, increasing brand visibility, generating potential leads, and driving traffic to your studio.

Lastly, it's essential to continuously monitor and evaluate the performance of your social media activities, analyzing metrics such as engagement, reach, and conversions. This helps identify what works well and what can be improved, allowing you to continuously adapt and optimize your social media promotion strategy to maximize the success of your nail technician studio.

4. Collaborations and Partnerships with Other Beauty Professionals

Collaborations and partnerships with other beauty professionals can be a valuable tool for expanding clientele and effectively promoting nail technician services. These synergies allow for offering integrated and combined packages that meet clients' beauty and wellness needs comprehensively and personalized.

A common strategy is to collaborate with estheticians, hairdressers, makeup artists, and other beauty professionals to offer combined packages that include nail technician services along with hair, face, and body treatments. This provides clients with a complete beauty and wellness experience, addressing their needs comprehensively and conveniently.

Partnerships with spas, wellness centers, and beauty salons can be particularly advantageous as they allow reaching a broader audience and offering services to clients who may not have been exposed to nail reconstruction practices before. Moreover, these collaborations can lead to increased client traffic through cross-referrals and joint promotions.

In addition to collaborations with other professionals, establishing partnerships with nail care product brands and cosmetics can provide visibility through promotional events, sponsorships, and endorsements. Such partnerships can help promote nail technician services and enhance credibility in the beauty industry.

Another collaboration opportunity is participating in beauty industry events and fairs, where professionals can meet, establish contacts, and create synergies for future collaborative projects and initiatives. Attending workshops, seminars, and training courses with other industry experts also offers valuable learning and professional growth opportunities.

Ultimately, collaborations and partnerships with other beauty professionals represent an important marketing and promotion strategy for nail technicians, allowing them to expand their client network, increase visibility, and add value to their services.

5. Special Offers and Loyalty Programs for Clients

Special offers and loyalty programs are powerful tools to incentivize clientele and effectively promote nail technician services. These initiatives are essential for creating a lasting bond with clients and encouraging them to return regularly for additional treatments.

Special offers can take various forms, including discounts on service prices, promotional packages that bundle multiple treatments at a reduced rate, and seasonal promotions tied to specific events such as Valentine's Day, Christmas, or birthdays. These offers are designed to attract new clients and stimulate interest among existing clients to try new treatments or services.

Loyalty programs are another effective strategy to reward regular clients and encourage their return. These programs may include points systems, where clients accumulate points each time they receive a treatment and can later redeem them for discounts or free treatments. Alternatively, they can offer exclusive benefits such as early access to new products or services, invitations to special events, and personalized gifts.

It is important to design special offers and loyalty programs that align with the needs and desires of your clientele. Therefore, conducting market research and surveys to better understand client preferences can help develop offers and programs that are enticing and relevant to them.

Furthermore, effectively communicating special offers and loyalty programs to clients through various communication channels, including websites, social media, newsletters, and promotional materials within your studio or salon, is crucial. Using engaging language and visually appealing graphics can help capture clients' attention and encourage them to participate in the offers and programs.

In conclusion, special offers and loyalty programs are valuable tools to promote nail technician services and incentivize clientele. Developing creative and personalized offers and programs can help build a stronger bond with clients and ensure long-term success for your business.

XXV. Conclusions and Future Perspectives

1. Summary of Key Topics Covered

This chapter aims to provide a comprehensive summary of the main topics covered throughout the book, with the goal of consolidating acquired knowledge and reinforcing understanding of fundamental concepts in the field of nail reconstruction using gel, acrylic, and polygel.

Throughout the learning journey, we have thoroughly explored each phase of the reconstruction process, starting from preparing the natural nail to the final refinement and polishing. We delved into the application techniques of different materials, analyzing their peculiarities and providing practical guidance to achieve optimal results.

Furthermore, we extensively discussed common issues and their respective solutions, offering valuable tips to tackle the most frequent challenges encountered in professional practice. Through practical examples, helpful advice, and advanced strategies, readers have had the opportunity to acquire solid skills and develop a thorough understanding of the nail technician profession.

In addition, the book also provided insights into marketing and promoting nail technician services, with targeted suggestions to reach and retain clientele.

In summary, the book has provided a comprehensive overview of the skills necessary to become a nail reconstruction professional, preparing the reader to successfully face challenges and opportunities in the field of hand beauty and wellness.

2. Reflections on the Evolution of the Nail Technician Industry

The nail technician industry has undergone significant evolution in recent years, influenced by a variety of factors that have shaped how nail care services are conceived and practiced. One of the most apparent transformations has been the advent of new technologies and innovative materials, which have revolutionized reconstruction techniques and expanded creative possibilities available to industry professionals.

The introduction of gel, acrylic, and polygel has opened new perspectives in nail reconstruction, allowing for increasingly natural, durable, and resilient results. Thanks to the versatility of these materials, complex designs, personalized shapes, and intricate decorations can be achieved, meeting diverse client needs and enabling nail technicians to express their creativity to the fullest.

Simultaneously, there has been a shift in consumer tastes and preferences, with growing attention to nail care and aesthetics. This has led to increased demand for professional services and a drive towards innovation within the industry, with constant updates to techniques and the introduction of new treatments aimed at improving nail health and appearance.

Furthermore, the rise of social media and digital platforms has revolutionized how nail care services are promoted and shared, providing industry professionals with new visibility opportunities and direct engagement with clients. An online presence has become essential for promoting work, showcasing results, and interacting with the audience in a direct and immediate manner.

In conclusion, the evolution of the nail technician industry has brought about profound changes in practices and professional perspectives, opening new paths and challenges for industry professionals. It is crucial for anyone working in this field to stay updated on the latest trends and innovations to consistently offer cutting-edge, high-quality services to their clientele.

3. Future Perspectives and Emerging Trends

Looking ahead to the future of the nail technician industry, several exciting perspectives and trends emerge that will influence how services are offered and professional activities conducted. One of the most significant trends is the heightened interest in sustainability and ecology, which is also reflected in the choice of materials and products used in nail reconstruction.

The use of biocompatible and environmentally low-impact materials will become increasingly prevalent, responding to growing consumer sensitivity towards environmental issues and the search for more eco-friendly solutions. Therefore, an increase in the use of natural and biodegradable products is expected, not only to meet market demands but also to adopt more sustainable practices in daily work.

Furthermore, there is a predicted further integration of digital technologies in the nail technician industry, with the development of innovative tools and applications for design visualization, client management, and service promotion. Augmented reality and virtual reality applications could become integral parts of the client experience, allowing previews of desired outcomes and maximizing service personalization.

Another emerging trend involves the expansion of nail care services beyond the traditional beauty salon context, including the creation of new business formats such as dedicated nail care studios, home services, and collaborations with other beauty industry professionals. This diversification of job opportunities offers new avenues for growth and development for industry operators, enabling them to reach a broader and more diverse clientele.

Finally, the importance of continuous education and professional development cannot be overstated in staying abreast of the latest industry trends and techniques. Continuous learning and acquiring new skills are essential to ensure high-quality performance and meet increasingly high client expectations.

In summary, the future perspectives of nail technology are characterized by a growing commitment to sustainability, technological innovation, service expansion, and high professionalism, which are key to success and growth in the industry.

4. Tips for Continuing to Grow and Adapt to Change

To continue growing and adapting to change in the nail technician industry, it is crucial to adopt a proactive approach focused on continuous learning. Here are some practical tips for industry operators looking to maintain their relevance and stay competitive in an ever-evolving market:

Professional Development: Invest in your education and participate in courses, workshops, and seminars to acquire new skills and stay abreast of the latest industry trends and technologies. Keeping your knowledge updated will enable you to offer innovative and high-quality services to your clients.

Experimentation and Research: Be open to experimentation and research into new techniques, materials, and products. Explore emerging trends and innovations in the industry and adapt them to your style and the needs of your clientele.

Networking: Attend industry events, beauty fairs, and meetings with other professionals to expand your network and share experiences and ideas. Networking can help you discover collaboration opportunities, gain valuable feedback and advice, and stay inspired by others' work.

Customer Feedback: Listen attentively to your customers' feedback and use it to improve your services and overall experience. Encourage them to express their opinions and preferences, and strive to meet their expectations as effectively as possible.

Adaptability: Be flexible and adaptable to market changes and customer demands. Observe emerging trends and customer requests, and adjust your business strategy and services accordingly to stay current.

Effective Marketing: Utilize effective marketing strategies to promote your services and reach new customers. Utilize social media, your website, local advertising, and other marketing platforms to increase your visibility and attract potential clients.

Maintaining Relationships: Cultivate lasting relationships with your existing customers by offering excellent service and maintaining regular contact through newsletters, special promotions, and other communication channels. Satisfied customers are key to obtaining recommendations and positive feedback.

Monitoring Results: Continuously monitor your business results and performance, analyzing metrics such as customer numbers, revenue, and satisfaction. Use this information to identify areas for improvement and plan your next steps.

By following these tips and maintaining an open, proactive attitude, you will be able to continue growing and adapting to the challenges and opportunities presented by the nail technician industry.

5. Acknowledgments and Conclusions

As we come to the conclusion of this manual dedicated to nail reconstruction with gel, acrylic, and polygel, I would like to express deep gratitude to all those who have made this project possible.

First and foremost, I would like to thank my collaborators who contributed their expertise and knowledge, offering invaluable advice and suggestions to ensure the quality and utility of this manual.

Special thanks go to all the professionals in the nail technician industry who generously shared their techniques and secrets, enriching the content of this book and making it a comprehensive and reliable resource for anyone wishing to learn and excel in this field.

I also want to express my gratitude to the readers who have shown interest and appreciation for this manual. Your support and feedback have been essential in guiding the creation of informative and practical content, tailored to meet your needs and questions.

Finally, I would like to thank my loved ones who supported and encouraged me throughout the writing process of this manual. Your moral and affectionate support was crucial in overcoming challenges and successfully completing this project.

In conclusion, I hope that this manual proves to be a useful resource for all those interested in learning nail reconstruction techniques with gel, acrylic, and polygel, and that it serves as a valuable tool for professional advancement in the field of nail technology. Thank you once again to everyone who made this journey of learning and growth possible.

Want one of our books for only $0.99? Here's how!

Hi there!
If you enjoyed this book, you can get your next title **for just $0.99**, choosing between:

📖 eBook
🖨 PDF of a print book

Follow these simple steps:

📍 **1.** Share your experience on the site where you purchased the book.

📍 **2.** Send a screenshot **of your feedback**, showing the "Verified Purchase" label, to:
info.testicreativi@gmail.com

📍 **3.** You'll receive a personal discount code to use in our online store, valid to get your next book **for only $0.99**.

📑 Your opinion truly matters: every feedback helps us grow and allows new readers to discover our books.

Thank you so much for your time, and happy reading!

www.ingramcontent.com/pod-product-compliance
Lightning Source LLC
Chambersburg PA
CBHW012301240726
48656CB00008B/2492